Lecture Notes in Medical Informatics

Lecture Notes in Medical Informatics

Edited by P. L. Reichertz and D. A. B. Lindberg

31

Stephen J. Duckett

Operations Research
for Health Planning
and Administration

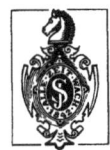

Springer-Verlag Berlin Heidelberg GmbH

Author

Stephen J. Duckett
Health Department Victoria
555 Collins Street
Melbourne, Victoria 3000, Australia

ISBN 978-3-540-17160-7   ISBN 978-3-642-93343-1 (eBook)
DOI 10.1007/978-3-642-93343-1

2127/3140-543210

TABLE OF CONTENTS

1   INTRODUCTION

Operations research aims to assist managers faced with problems of coordinating activities; improving the quality of care of services delivered; making optimal resource allocation decisions and generally, managing services and institutions. Operations research (or O.R.) was originally developed in response to the problems of the second World War. It was characterised then by a unifying and clear objective; clear problems that had to be solved and the use of inter-disciplinary teams to analyse and solve identified problems. This analysis often drew on mathematical techniques.

After the war, operations research moved in two separate but related directions. In England, the emphasis on inter-disciplinary approaches and problem solving teams remained. The operations researcher still used mathematical techniques but these were not systematised into a volume of standard formulae. The emphasis of operations research was on the _approach_ not the _tools_ used (see, for example, Luckman & Stringer, 1974; also Luck, Luckman, Smith & Stringer 1971; and McLachlan, 1975).

In the United States, the emphasis was placed on the use of mathematical techniques. Operations research became a mathematically based science relying on standardised models (e.g. queuing, allocation) and formulae. This approach was facilitated by the availability of computers.

Both approaches to operations research have a lot to offer. It is useful to be able to model problems mathematically and formulate optimal solutions but, obviously, the problems managers face can rarely be fitted into one of the "pure" operations research problem types. The analysis of the problem under consideration might thus benefit from the more reflective British approach. In a sense, of course, this UK-US dichotomy is a caricature of the approaches adopted in both countries and there is certainly evidence that attention is being paid in the US to the (UK) problem solving basis (Ackoff 1979a, 1979b). This synthesis reflects two important points. First, problems faced by managers are complex and that a useful starting point for any analysis is to "model" the system under review using mathematical techniques. Secondly, there are common problems and approaches that can be systematised into operations research problem types to which standard approaches and analytical techniques can be applied. We will be examining a number of those major problem types e.g. inventory problems, queuing problems etc. But first, it is useful to highlight the use of models in operations research.

THE USE OF MODELS

Organisations are complex arrangements of people, machinery and systems and a manager's job is to facilitate the operation of the various parts of an organisation and to plan for future development. Managers cannot be expected to be completely familiar with every aspect of every part of the organisation in which they are working, but they must be able to co-ordinate the disparate parts. All organisations are comprised of a myriad of inter-relating parts and a manager should attempt to take into account the full ramifications of any decision he or she makes.

A manager thus has to simplify the operations of his or her organisation so that it can be understood. March and Simon (1958) have suggested that humans suffer from 'bounded' or 'limited' rationality. They suggest that modern organisations are so complex and the information requirements so great that humans can never hope to be fully cognisant of all the ramifications of decisions. They argue (p.130):

> "The organisational and social environment in which the decision maker finds himself determines what consequences he will anticipate, what ones he will not; what alternatives he will consider, what ones he will ignore. In a theory of organisation these variables cannot be treated as unexplained independent factors, but must themselves be determined and predicted by the theory...choice is always exercised with respect to a limited, approximate, simplified 'model' of the real situation...the chooser's....definition of the situation."

Managers, therefore, will implicitly build models to assist their understanding of complex issues. It should be remembered, however that models are used to simplify complex issues, not to isolate problems from their environment.

Modelling of relationships and structures will, without doubt, be increasingly used in health service administration and planning. Forrester (1961, p.49) states:

> "Models have become widely accepted as a means for studying complex phenomena. A model is a substitute for some real equipment or system. The value of a model arises from its improving our understanding of obscure behaviour characteristics more effectively than could be done by observing the real system. A model, compared to the real system it represents, can yield information at lower cost. Knowledge can be obtained more quickly and for conditions not observable."

Many different types of models exist, each with their different characteristics, their different uses and their different advantages. These models differ in their level of "abstraction", from physical models (or mock-ups) as the least abstract to mathematical models as the most abstract. Operations research generally relies on the development of a mathematical model of the system being studied.

Mathematical models can be subdivided into two main types: deterministic and probabilistic. The simpler type is the deterministic model. This type is one wherein variables take only specified values. The second type is the probabilistic model which recognises that we often cannot know the actual values that variables will take, and so probabilities are assigned to the different values, and these are used in the model. Thus, for example, you cannot say that a person will turn up at a hospital in a given five minute period but you can assign a probability of an arrival (often based on historic data). Probabilistic models are also known as 'stochastic' models: stochastic means 'governed by the laws of probability' and is taken from a Greek word meaning 'aim it' or 'guess'.

Model building (especially mathematical model building) is the essence of operations research. The models of operations research are mainly concerned with relations of the form $P = f(C_i, U_i)$ were P is a measure of the overall performance of the system,

C_i represents the set of controllable variables (eg C_1, C_2, C_3, C_4...) and

U_i represents the set of variables regarded as uncontrollable in this model (eg U_1, U_2...) and

f   defines the relationship i.e. we are saying that the performance of the system is some function of the interaction of the controllable and uncontrollable variables.

Thus we can see the three basic elements of all decision making:

<u>Uncontrollable variables</u>, which can be defined as those factors in a system or its environment that are beyond the decision-maker's control even though they may affect the outcome of the decision. Examples of uncontrollable variables include the weather, prevailing morbidity patterns and, for models used by some agencies, government policy.

<u>Controllable variables</u>, which are defined as those variables under the decision-makers' control (e.g. number of hospital beds, their distribution (whether medical or surgical), staffing patterns) and can either be those variables which can be varied in the future (the site of a new hospital) or those variables which can be varied in the present time period (within certain limits, staff allocation). The two types of controllable variables are sometimes known as planning and operating variables respectively. Importantly, variables which are uncontrollable in the short run, might be controllable when modelling over a longer time horizon. Similarly variables which are uncontrollable in a model developed for use by a hospital, might be controllable when included in a model developed for use by a health planning authority.

Outcome or <u>performance</u> variables are those variables which give a quantification of the degree to which the system has achieved its objectives.

Problems with Modelling

Many people use models every day without realising that they do
so! A commonly used model is an 'Ability to Pay Model' (often
called a 'Means Test') Such a model is normally of the form:

    N = Y - (R+cD)
where
N = Net Income for purpose of test Y = Weekly Income
    R = Rent
    c = Constant
    D = No. of dependents.

    If N is less than A a patient may be defined as eligible for a
    benefit under social security arrangements.

This model is, of course, very simple to apply. One problem
involved in the use of such a model is, however, that the variables
used may not be relevant or may need modification. Let us assume
that the model measures what society regards as a persons ability to
pay their medical and/or hospital bills. The most commonly used
value for weekly income will be the income prior to admission; but
that may have little relation to income after discharge which will
be an important factor in determining ability to pay!

Similarly the age of the dependents and whether they are twins would
probably also affect ability to pay. Clearly to get a more accurate
and reliable estimate one should take into account a host of extra
variables.

        N = Y' - (R+f(D))
        Y'= Probable net income after discharge
        f (D) = a function concerning the number of dependents and
        their ages, the number of multiple births etc.

This model is more complicated and a difficult one to use. This
situation is illustrative of one of the problems involved in the use
of models: a model has to be simple enough to be understood and
easily used yet complex enough to represent reality adequately.

This fundamental tradeoff between simplicity (and ease of use) and
complexity (and more relevance but at a higher cost of development)
is common to most operations research applications and, indeed, this
will be seen in the ensuing discussion of operations research
problem types. Our discussion of inventory models for example, will
commence with a simple model which is easy to use and we will relax
some of the assumptions to move to a more complex, more useful but
more costly model.

STEPS IN OPERATIONS RESEARCH

Warner & Holloway (1978), identify four steps in any use
of operations research:

1. Problem and Model Formulation
2. Quantification
3. Solution
4. Sensitivity Analysis.

Implementing these steps involves elements of judgement on the part of the model builder and assumptions that may or may not be justified. Users of operations research should continually question all the assumptions made - whether they are explicit or implicit.

Step 1: Problem and Model Formulation

The first step to be undertaken is to model the decision. Warner & Holloway (1978, p12) suggest that most decisions that managers make fall into three categories:

> Resource-Size Decisions - choosing the amount of resources to provide in order to meet demand. In most cases, the decision is how much demand to meet or, more to the point, how much _not_ to meet.

> Procedure Decisions - _given_ a level of demand to meet, choosing the best (usually lowest cost) way to meet it.

> Scheduling Decisions - choosing the arrangement or manipulation of a _given_ level of resources and/or a _given_ level of demand to best meet objectives.

They also point out that management involves a _control problem_ defined as:

> choosing measures of performance for monitoring systems and, when necessary, choosing among the above three decisions (in addition to organizational design alternatives) such that systems continue to achieve objectives.

The classification of a problem or decision is part of the early stages of the analysis process. Warner & Holloway also define certain other stages of this problem and model formulation step and these are listed below (together with some questions that should be asked):

(i)   identify the system objectives
        (Have they identified the right ones?)

(ii)   identify the different options available
        (Have they identified the full range of options?)

(iii)   identify the constraints
        (Have they identified all the constraints; are the levels of the constraints realistic?)

(iv)   establish measures of performance for each objective
        (Are they appropriate?)

Warner & Holloway rightly point out that it is at the problem and model formulation stage that the primary responsibility of health administrators lies. It is important to recall here March and Simon's comments quoted above (p2) about bounded rationality: can we consider all the options, all the constraints?

Step 2: Quantification

Having formulated the model, the next step is to quantify it. Again assumptions are involved and administrators should be wary of them: is the time period chosen for assessing benefits adequate; are the assessments of cost-savings realistic (they are almost always exagerated); what about non-quantified items?

Step 3: Solution

Having undertaken the quantification stage, the problem is posed for solution. This involves comparison of the options, identification of optimal strategies etc.

Step 4: Sensitivity Analysis

The final step in the operations research process is sensitivity analysis. This is again an area in which the health administrator will play an important role. It is at this step that the administrator brings together all the earlier comments about assumptions of the study, plus the possibility of errors. As Warner & Holloway put it (p29):

> "(T)here comes a time when we must face the question of how much the compromises made in the quantification affect the quality of the result of the analysis (the decision)."

We need to assess the impact of varying certain assumptions and varying the values of key variables.

Operations Research or What?

The use of operations research in health administration poses a number of problems:

> It involves quantification, but how much should we quantify?

> How can operations research techniques be used when many things cannot be quantified?

> What is the role of the health administrator who is not an operations research specialist?

Of course it is recognised managers do not and could not use operations research techniques to assist with every decision, but an increased use of rational decision making is essential if we are to achieve a more efficient health care system. Lindblom (1959) compares what he suggests are two alternative methods of decision making.

Rational-Comprehensive	Successive Limited Comparisons
1a. Clarification of values or objectives distinct from and usually prerequisite to empirical analysis of alternative policies.	1b. Selection of values goals and empirical analysis of the needed action are not distinct from one another but are closely intertwined.
2a. Policy-formulation is approached through means-end analysis: first the ends are isolated, then the means to achieve them are sought.	2b. Since means and ends are distinct, means-end analysis is often inappropriate or limited.
3a. The test of a 'good' policy is that it can be shown to be the most appropriate means to desired ends.	3b. The test of a 'good' policy is typically that various analysts find themselves directly agreeing on a policy (without their agreeing that it is the most appropriate means to an agreed objective).
4a. Analysis is comprehensive, every important relevant factor is taken into account.	4b. Analysis is drastically limited: i) Important alternative potential policies are neglected. ii) Important possible consequences are neglected. iii) Important affected values are neglected.
5a. Theory is often heavily relied upon.	5b. A succession of comparisons greatly reduces or eliminates reliance on theory."

Lindblom argues that successive limited comparison is the most commonly used method and, indeed, this cannot be denied. Lindblom does not see this as an ideal method, his point is simply to describe reality. It is clear however that better decisions are made by the rational-comprehensive method, we should therefore try to enhance it use and it is here that operations research has a role to play.

Operations Research in Health Planning & Administration

Application of operations research to health planning and administration is increasing dramatically and the last decade has seen a number of publications reviewing the 'state of the art'. (see especially Fries, 1981; Stimson & Stimson, 1972; Shuman, Speas & Young, 1975. Shorter reviews include Palmer, 1975; Papageorgiou, 1978; Duncan & Currow, 1978). An indication of the growth in the literature can be seen by comparing the bibliography by Dunaye, Foote & Dunaye (1971) with those of Fries (1976, 1979). Some introductory texts dealing with aspects of operations research and health administration have been prepared by Griffith (1972), Warner & Holloway (1978), Relsman (1979), Wren (1974) & Koza (1973). A number of book length reports of specialised health related operations research studies have also been published e.g. a linear programming study in Dowling (1976); a queuing and simulation study in Rising (1977) and a discussion of applications of inventory models in Ammer (1975).

These notes are designed to supplement those other works and to provide a comprehensive introduction to the major operations research types. The examples are all drawn from health administration and planning problems.

CONCLUSION

The use of operations research implies a recognition of the fact that all parts of an organisation are related and are interacting. Operations research, however, simplifies problems by modelling the problem in mathematical terms. The model can then be used by managers to assist them in planning and decision making.

REFERENCES

Ackoff, R.L. (1979a) "The Future of Operational Research is Past" Journal of the Operational Research Society, Vol. 30, No. 2, (February) pp.93-104.

Ackoff, R.L. (1979b) "Resurrecting the Future of Operational Research" Journal of the Operational Research Society, Vol. 30, No. 3, (March), pp.189-200.

Ammer, D.S. (1975) Purchasing & Materials Management for Health Care Institutions, Lexington.

Boldy, D. & Clayden, D. (1979) "Operational Research Projects in Health & Welfare Services in the United Kingdom & Ireland" Journal of the Operational Research Society, Vol. 30, No. 6, (June), pp.505-512.

Dowling, W.L. (1976) Hospital Production: A Linear Programming Model, Lexington.

Dunaye, T.M., Foote, B.C. & Dunaye, S.L. (1971) "Health Planning Applications of Operations Research & Systems Analysis" Council of Planning Librarian Exchange Bibliography, 233, (November).

Forrester, J.W. (1961) Industrial Dynamics, Wiley.

Fries, B.E. (1981) Applications of Operations Research to Health Care Delivery Systems: A Complete Review of the Periodical Literature, (Lecture Notes in Medical Informatics No. 10) Springer Verlag.

Griffith, J.R. (1972) Quantitative Techniques for Hospital Planning and Control, Heath.

Koza, R.L. (1973) Mathematical and Operations Research Techniques in Health Administration, Colorado Assoc. UP.

Lindblom, C.E. (1959) "The Science of 'Muddling Through" Public Administrative Review, Vol. XIX, No. 1 (Winter), pp.79-88.

Luckman, J. & Stringer, J. (1974) "The Operational Research Approach to Problem Solving" _Britlsh Medical Bulletin_, Vol. 30 No. 3, pp.257-261.

Luck, G.M., Luckman, J., Smith, B. & Stringer, J. (1971) _Patients, Hospitals and Operational Research_, Tavistock.

March, J.G. & Simon, H.A. (1958) _Organizations_, Wiley.

McLachlan, G. (1975) _Measuring for Management - Quantitative Methods in Health Service Management_, Oxford UP.

Reisman, A. (1979) _Systems Analysis in Health-Care Delivery_, Lexington.

Rising, E.J. (1977) _Ambulatory Care Systems Vol. 1: Design for Improved Patient Flow_, Lexington.

Shuman, L.J. et al (1976) _Operations Research in Health Care: A Critical Analysis_, Johns Hopkins UP.

Stimson, D.H. & Stimson, R.H. (1972) _Operations Research in Hospitals: Diagnosis and Prognosis_, Hospital Research & Education Trust.

Wren, G.R. (1974) _Modern Health Administration_, Georgia UP.

Warner, D.M. & Holloway, D.C. (1978) _Decision Making & Control for Health Administration: The Management of Quantitative Analysis_, Health Administration Press.

2   INVENTORIES

How many units of drug A should be held in the pharmacy? How much cleaning fluid should be stored in the central store? How many beds should a new hospital have? Although these questions deal with a variety of situations they have one thing in common, they can all be modelled as "inventory" problems. The typical problem can be posed simply: how much of given item should be held in stock. That simplicity, however, masks a range of extensions and appliations. First, however, a definition of inventory: an inventory can be defined as a store of resources standing idle awaiting use. The most obvious hospital inventories are the items held in the general store and the items in the pharmacy department. In both these cases items are held in the inventories for later use within the hospital. But the definition adopted allows for a wider application of inventory models: empty beds in Ward X, trainee medical technologists (who are supernumery during training) and money in the bank are all examples of inventories. These empty beds, trainees and dollars are idle awaiting use. The provision of the beds and the salaries of the trainees are costs to the hospital and the community and whilst they are idle, the community gets no return.

The elements of inventory models

All inventories have certain common elements. These include costs, demand patterns and order patterns.

There are two major types of costs involved in holding inventories:

1.   Costs involved in holding the inventory and

2.   Costs involved in not holding the inventory. (or, more precisely, costs involved in holding only a specific level of inventory).

With the first type of cost, the larger the average size of the inventory, the greater will be the expense. Typical costs of this type are depreciation, insurance, cost of capital tied up in holding the stocks etc. The second type of cost is rather different. In this case, the smaller the average inventory, the larger will be the cost. This type of cost typically includes costs associated with not having an item in stock when it is needed, the cost of emergency ordering and so on. However, it can quickly be seen that the cost of placing the ordinary order for goods would also be of this type since if the average inventory is only small, orders would have to be placed for replenishment stock at frequent intervals, thus increasing the cost!

The major problem addressed by inventory models is to find the balance between the two types of costs to arrive at the optimal level of inventory.

In addition to these costs, inventory models have two other major elements: the demand patterns and order patterns. The number of items in an inventory at any given time obviously depends on the demand for those items. Obviously if there is a high demand items will be removed from the inventory frequently and it will run down quickly. In most organisations, management cannot greatly affect the demand for items and so in most inventory models, including those discussed herein, demand is assumed to be an uncontrollable variable.

On the other hand, management can control the number of orders placed throughout the year - it can further affect the size of the inventory by varying the number of items acquired with each order. Thus elements of the ordering pattern can clearly be seen to be controllable variables.

Let us now look in more detail at the two types of costs associated with inventories.

1. <u>Procurement Costs or Order Costs</u>

These consist of all those expenses involved with the acquisition of goods for the inventory. These costs include such items as the clerical costs associated with the ordering goods (making out requisitions etc.), the costs associated with paying the bill for the goods as well as certain costs in the store such as updating the inventory record, uncrating and inspecting the goods purchased. It can be assumed that order costs do not vary significantly with the size of order placed. For example, the costs of paying a bill are the same whether the bill is for $10 or $10,000. When certain costs do not vary with the amount ordered, they are said to be 'independent' of the amount ordered.

2. <u>Stockage Costs and Holding Costs</u>

These are the costs associated with actually holding items in an inventory. Three main types of stockage costs can be distinguished.

(i) Carrying Costs

These include the direct costs associated with holding an inventory - included here would be such items as insurance premiums, air conditioning or refrigeration charges, security costs associated with the warehouse. A major cost which is included is the cost of having capital "tied up" in inventories (rather than investing it elsewhere).

Another type of carrying cost is the cost associated with the deterioration or depreciation of goods held. For example, if stationery is held for long periods it will turn yellow and will not be able to be used - this deterioration is a slow process and, over many thousands of items, can be ascribed a value.

(ii) Overstock Costs

Despite the most careful planning, items occasionally remain which are unusable after meeting current demand. The classic example is the stock of Christmas trees remaining after Christmas Day. An example familiar to most hospital staff would be the stock of medicinals not used by the expiry date.

(iii) 'Out of Stock' Costs

Occasionally items are demanded from an inventory when there is no stock to satisfy the demand. When the level of inventory is zero, stock-out costs are incurred. Inventory models normally treat these in one of two ways:

(a) Back ordering

It can be assumed that goods not held can be 'back ordered', i.e., the customer's order will be filed and, when the next delivery is received, the customer's order will be met. The costs associated with this sort of transaction include loss of goodwill and costs associated with expediting delivery of items (e.g. hiring a taxi to ensure delivery, cost penalties imposed by the supplier, extra shipping and handling costs).

(b) Lost sales

In the lost sales case, it is assumed that the customer is thoroughly disgusted and transfers allegiance to another supplier. In this case as well as the loss of goodwill there is an opportunity cost measured by the failure to make a sale and the lost profit associated with that.

Clearly, the more items that are held in an inventory, the greater will be the stockage costs. Conversely, the more items held in an inventory, the smaller will be the number of orders placed and hence the lower the order costs.

Measurement of Costs

An optimal solution to the inventory problem depends on establishing an 'inventory model' of a mathematical nature. This model involves establishing the relationship between the level of inventory held and the total cost - the measurement of these costs may be the most difficult aspect of the determination of an inventory model.

Obviously measuring these costs requires detailed cost accounting type data. Some of the relevant cost components, for example direct storage costs, may be determined directly from the organization's records. In other cases, especially in respect of loss of 'goodwill', no relevant records are likely to be available. It would therefore be necessary to rely on the opinions of the managers about the magnitudes of these costs. A particular manager may be asked what he or she would pay to avoid one unit being out of stock for the item in question. The resulting inventory decisions will at least be consistent with the manager's opinion. It also turns out however that in most cases the optimum stock position is not changed very much even by large errors in the measurement of costs.

When all the costs are added, inventories can be quite expensive. Order costs quickly mount up when one includes the accounting department's time in drawing cheques and bank charges, on top of the costs of the clerical staff in placing and recording orders. Similarly, stockage costs are surprisingly expensive.

A study of carrying costs in a hospital in Iowa with an $82,000 investment in inventory showed that carrying costs were approximately a third of the total value of the inventory (See Table 2.1 taken from Ammer 1975, p.91. A more detailed discussion of costs associated with inventories can be found in Ammer 1975, pp.85-95). Since that study was undertaken there have been increases in both salaries and wages and interest rates and so the total costs and the proportion of costs to the total value of the inventory are likely to be much higher.

Table 2.1   Actual Carrying Costs of an Iowa Hospital with an $82,000 Investment in Inventory.

Category	Annual Cost	Cost as a Percent of Inventory
Salaries	$6,913	8.4%
Depreciation	4,000	4.9
Insurance	500	0.6
Repairs	1,000	1.2
Utilities	1,000	1.2
Total Stores	$13,413	16.3%
Shrinkage	$4,400	5.4
Obsolescence	2,000	2.4
Total Losses	$6,400	7.8%
8% Interest	6,560	8.0
Total Carrying Cost	$26,373	32.1%

A final point when considering inventories which requires considerable emphasis is that the problem of determining the optimum level of stocks in always present and it should not be ignored simply because costs may be difficult to measure. Whatever course of action is taken (based perhaps on guesswork or "intuition") imputes a value to the ratio of the opposing costs. It may be that the value thus imputed for the loss of goodwill "cost", for example, may be excessively high in relation to other costs. Indeed empirical studies of "rule of thumb" inventory policies have revealed this situation - organisations often tend to hold excessively large stocks of items because of a mistaken belief that they should never run the risk of being "out of stock". In fact, unless out of stock costs are infinitely large, the optimum policy will involve occasions when stocks are exhausted.

INVENTORY MODELS

Many different types of inventory models have been formulated and
most of the situations faced by managers have now been modelled.
Just as methods for controlling inventories vary, so do inventory
models. It will be recalled that one of the three major
components of inventory models is the order pattern. Most
inventory models are based on order point systems. These are
systems where the order quantity is fixed and an order is placed
whenever stock reaches a certain level (the order point). We
will be concentrating on these types of systems. The other major
type of system is the order period system which allows the order
quantity to fluctuate but establishes a fixed interval or time
period when the stock of every item in the inventory is reviewed
and orders placed as required.

Models of order point systems focus on two major variables: the
reorder point and the order quantity. Order quantity may be
dfined as the number of items placed in any order or group of
orders. The reorder point is that level of inventory where we
automatically place the order. A further term used is lead time
which is defined as the delay between placing an order and its
receipt.

The various types of inventory models can be classified according
to realism, complexity or any number of other variables. It is
reasonable to assume, however, that the more realistic a model
is, the more complicated it is mathematically. We will deal with
only three of the models that have been developed – one where
demand is assumed to be known with certainty and two where a
probability distribution is used to predict future demand. The
three models discussed are in order of both increasing realism
and increasing complexity.

DETERMINISTIC MODEL

The deterministic model is the simplest inventory model and
includes a number of simplifying assumptions. Briefly it models
a situation where demand for items from the inventory is known
with certainty and we are attempting to identify what size
inventory we should hold. In terms of our contollable variables
we must either decide how often an order should be placed or how
large an order should be placed (or a combination of the two).

The deterministic model involves the following assumptions:

(a) Demand is known and is uniform (i.e. steady) throughout
the whole period concerned.

(b) Reordering takes place when the stock reaches a
particular level and the delay involved in delivery of
new stock is constant. Since the "lead time" is
constant, as is the rate of demand, we can set our
reorder point equal to the demand during lead time and
be certain that goods will be received in time to
ensure that we can meet any demands on the inventory.

(c) Procurement costs and carrying costs are known. (Since
demand and supply are known with certainty we can also

assume that 'out of stock' and 'over stock' costs are zero.)

(d)   Orders have to be placed in specified (unchangeable) sizes, e.g. if we decide to order in batches of 76, this size cannot be changed so that the next order is for 78 etc., thus we are assuming there is a <u>fixed re-order quantity</u>.

Since we have fixed the reorder point in assumption (b), we have now reduced the inventory problem to determining the optimum order quantity.

Let us assume that we are determining the inventory policy for the year and define the variables with which we are concerned as follows:

Q = number of items in each order (sometimes called the Economic Order Quantity (EOQ) or Reorder Quantity)

A = number of inventory items demanded per year (which is also the number of units to be supplied)

C = aggregate (Total) cost per annum

C_1 = procurement cost <u>per order placed</u> (in dollars)

C_2 = carrying cost <u>per unit of inventory</u> held for the year (in dollars)

N = number of orders placed per year

R = reorder point

The optimum order quantity will be that level of Q for which C (Total Cost) is minimised. Now since we assumed stockout costs and overstock costs were zero we know that

Total Cost = Procurement cost plus Carrying cost

Let us now determine the size of each of these costs.

Order or Procurement Cost

The total annual procurement cost will simply be the procurement cost of each order multiplied by the number of orders:

Total procurement cost = $C_1 N$

But we still have to determine the value of N.

If we are running our inventory efficiently, the number of orders placed must be such that we can satisfy the total demand. The total number of units supplied is obviously the number of orders placed multiplied by the size of each order, and this should thus equal the total number of units demanded:

i.e. $A = Q \times N$

and hence $N = \dfrac{A}{Q}$

and hence, substituting, total procurement cost $= C_1 \dfrac{A}{Q}$

Carrying cost

Carrying costs can be calculated quite simply by multiplying the average number of items held in stock by the carrying cost of each item. Although we know the second term of the multiplication (C_2), we still must calculate the average inventory. Figure 2.1 shows how the level of a typical deterministic inventory might fluctuate over the year.

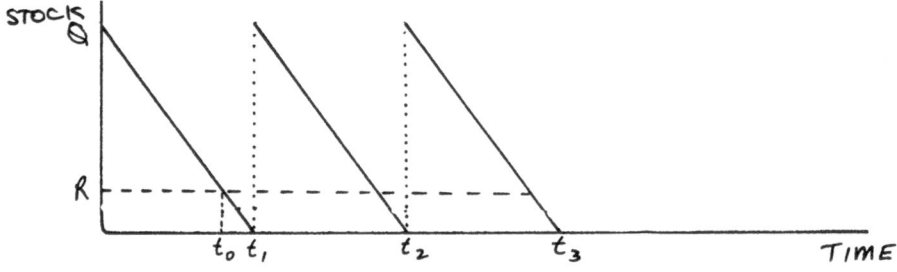

Figure 2.1

If we assume the year starts with Q goods in stock, they are slowly depleted over time until the reorder point (R) is reached and a new order placed. After lead time $(t_1 - t_0)$, the level of inventory reaches zero and a new shipment arrives of size Q. This usage-replacement cycle then continues over the whole year.

Now, we are interested in determining the average amount of inventory held. Since the average in each time period is clearly the same we shall merely look at the first time period. Now at the start of the first time period there were Q units in stock and these were steadily depleted so that at the end of the period there were zero units left. The average level of inventory is obviously going to be the mean of these two values.

Hence average inventory $= \dfrac{\text{initial inventory} + \text{closing inventory}}{2}$

$$= \frac{Q + 0}{2}$$

$$= \frac{Q}{2}$$

Since we know that carrying cost is the average inventory multiplied by the carring cost per unit of inventory held:

total carrying cost $= C_2 \dfrac{Q}{2}$

Recalling that total inventory cost is the sum of carrying cost and procurement cost, we can now formulate an equation for the total inventory cost per year:

$$C = C_1 \frac{A}{Q} + C_2 \frac{Q}{2}$$

It can be shown that total costs are minimised when procurement cost is equal to carrying cost* and hence the optimum order quantity is at that value of Q where

$$C_1 \frac{A}{Q} = C_2 \frac{Q}{2}$$

Which can easily be found:

$$C_1 A = \frac{C_2 Q^2}{2} \qquad \text{(multiplying both sides by Q)}$$

$$2C_1 A = C_2 Q^2 \qquad \text{(multiplying both sides by 2)}$$

$$\frac{2C_1 A}{C_2} = Q^2 \qquad \text{(dividing both sides by } C_2\text{)}$$

$$Q = \sqrt{\frac{2C_1 A}{C_2}} \qquad \text{(taking the square root of both sides)}$$

and thus we have found the economic (optimum) order quantity.**

Thus the optimum order size can be easily determined if procurement costs, carrying costs and the total demand are known.

---

*   By use of calculus, $\frac{dC}{dQ} = 0$ when C is minimised.

$$\frac{dC}{dQ} = \frac{-C_1 A}{Q^2} + \frac{C_2}{2}$$

$$= 0 \text{ when } \frac{C_2}{2} = \frac{C_1 A}{Q^2}$$

$$Q^2 = \frac{2C_1 A}{C_2}$$

** Other formulae are also available. Warner and Holloway (1978), p.63), for instance use the following formula:

$$Q = \sqrt{\frac{2CU}{w + ip}}$$

This formula essentially provides an expanded form for the estimation of C_2.

It is important to note that all three affect the optimum order size - not just the total demand. Logically, the higher the procurement costs (C_1) the higher will be the optimum order size (and hence the lower the total procurement costs) and the higher the carrying costs, the lower the optimum order size. As you should also note that the relationship is not direct (a square root is taken), and so there should be some scope for economies of scale.

Example 2.1

A hospital uses 10,000 packets of bandages per annum, and the rate of usage is constant throughout the year. It has been determined that the procurement cost per order is $25 and the carrying costs amnount to 12.5¢ per packet of bandages held.

$$
\begin{aligned}
\text{Clearly } A &= 10,000 \\
C_1 &= \$25 \\
C_2 &= \$0.125
\end{aligned}
$$

$$
\begin{aligned}
Q &= \sqrt{\frac{2C_1 A}{C_2}} \\
&= \sqrt{\frac{2 \times 25 \times 10,000}{\frac{125}{1000}}} \\
&= \sqrt{\frac{2 \times 10,000,000}{5}} \\
&= \sqrt{4,000,000} \\
&= 2,000
\end{aligned}
$$

Hence orders should be placed in lots of 2,000.

Other values that can be determined are:

(i) Average size of inventory $= \dfrac{Q}{2}$

$$= \frac{2,000}{2}$$

$$= 1,000 \text{ items}$$

(ii) Number of orders to be placed $= \dfrac{A}{Q}$

$$= \frac{10,000}{2,000}$$

$$= 5$$

(iii) Number of days between orders $= \dfrac{365}{5}$

$$= 73 \text{ days}$$

The costs associated with various order quantities can be seen in the following table:

Table 2.2

Order Quantity Q	Procurement Costs $C_1\frac{A}{Q}$	Holding Costs $C_2\frac{Q}{2}$	Total Costs C
500	500.00	31.25	531.25
750	333.33	46.88	380.21
1,000	250.00	62.50	312.50
1,250	200.00	78.13	278.13
1,500	166.67	93.75	260.42
1,750	142.86	109.38	252.24
2,000	125.00	125.00	250.00
2,250	111.11	140.63	251.74
2,500	100.00	156.25	256.25
2,750	90.91	171.88	262.79
3,000	83.33	187.50	270.83

It is interesting to note the wide variation in total costs (from $531.25 to $250. p.a.). These costs can be plotted as follows and the relationship between minimum total cost and the intersection of holding costs and procurement costs seen at a glance:

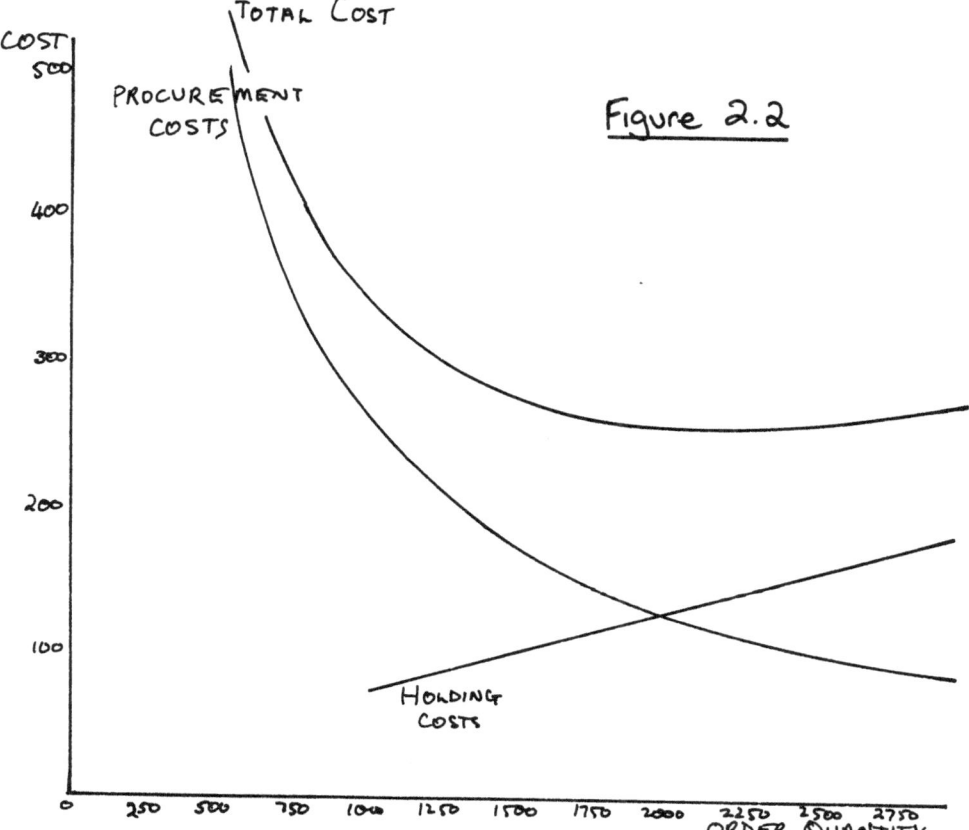

Figure 2.2

PROBABILISTIC MODEL

The second type of inventory model is one which allows for an element of random variations. This type of model is sometimes called 'stochastic' after the greek word for 'aim' or 'marksman'.

The deterministic model reflected a situation where demand was known with certainty and the lead time could also be accurately predicted - this situation is often a long way from reality! If we allow demand and lead time to fluctuate randomly we can utilise two different approaches in an attempt to pursue an optimum inventory policy:

> (a) we could attempt to generate a mathematical model (similar to the deterministic model) to specify precisely all the costs and thus determine the optimum inventory policy

or (b) we could simply rely on a 'buffer stock' to attempt to cope with fluctuation in demand.

The assumptions involved in both models are similar:

> (a) Total demand for the year is known but daily (weekly or monthly) demand is not known with certainty. However a probability distribution can be deduced (from past experience) for use in the model.

> (b) Reordering takes place when the stock reaches a particular level but the delay between placing an order and its receipt may be subject to random variation and so a probability distribution is also associated with the lead time.

> (c) Procurement costs and carrying costs are known. Overstock costs are zero. Stockouts may occur and they are met by backordering.

> (d) There is a fixed reorder quantity.

Our initial 'saw tooth' diagram for inventory usage thus becomes more like Figure 2.3.

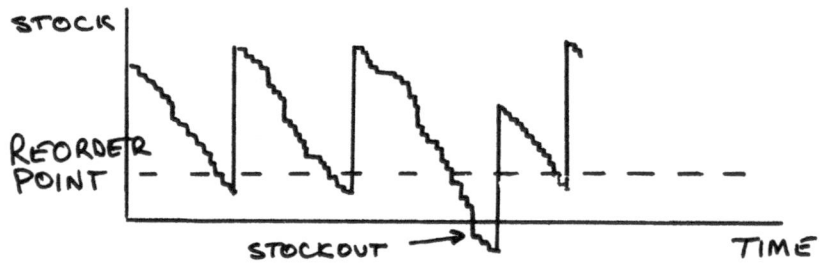

Figure 2.3

There are two major factors which will determine whether or not stocks are exhausted: the length of the lead time and the demand on each of the lead-time days. Thus the simultaneous occurrence of an abnormally high demand and an unusually large lead time would tend to produce a 'stockout'.

Both the mathematical and the buffer stock models take account of stockouts. Both of them also differ from the deterministic model in that they use two variables to define the optimum inventory policy: order quantity and reorder point. In the deterministic model, the reorder point was set equal to lead time whereas in the probabilistic approaches the reorder point is a variable to be manipulated.

Let us now consider the buffer stock approach to solving situations where demand and lead time are assumed to be stochastic.

Buffer Stocks

Essentially the buffer stock model that we will examine assumes that you have used the deterministic model to arrive at an optimum order quantity. (You will recall that this value does not depend on the reorder point or lead time.) The second step is to determine the optimum reorder point which will have to cater for both variations in demand and variations in the lead time. We can start by establishing the minimum level at which the reorder point can safely be set. Obviously the reorder point must be at least as large as the average demand during lead time and preferably, somewhat larger than this to cope with fluctuations in both lead time and demand. This excess is termed the buffer stock.

Recalling the variables that were defined earlier and letting

$$B = \text{Buffer Stock,}$$

$$D = \text{Average Demand during lead time}$$

then $R = D + B$

The decision on the level of the reorder point is still not a simple one for the larger the buffer stock is made, the smaller will be the probability that a stockout will occur but, of course, the larger the buffer stock is, the larger will be the amount of capital tied up.

The calculation of R in a Buffer Stock Model

Average demand during lead time depends on both the number of units demanded per day or other unit of time and the length of the lead time. In fact, average (or, more precisely, expected) demand during lead time is the product of expected demand per day and expected lead time. Thus if u = expected (average) demand per day
b = expected (average) lead time
then D = u b

Recalling that the expected value of an event which has a number of possible outcomes is simply the sum of the value of each outcome multiplied by the respective probability:

By definiton $u = \sum_i p_i i$

where p_i = probability that i units are
demanded on any day

and $b = \sum_j p_j j$

where p_j = probability of a lead time of
j days

Example 2.2

Let us assume that the demand per day and the lead time for a
certain drug used by a hospital can be defined in terms of the
probability distrbution shown in Table 2.3.

Table 2.3 Demand and Supply of Drug

DRUG DEMAND

Units demanded/day	Probability of specified demand
0	.4
1	.3
2	.2
3	.1
	1.0

LEAD TIME FOR SUPPLY OF DRUGS

Lead Time (in days)	Probability of Specified Lead Time
1	.25
2	.5
3	.25
	1.0

The expected demand during lead time is given by

$$D = u\ b$$

The expected demand per day, u, is the sum of the number of units
demanded multiplied by the probability of that level of demand.

$u = (0 \times .4) + (1 \times .3) + (2 \times .2) + (3 \times .1)$
$= 0 + .3 + .4 + .3$
$= 1.0$

The expected lead time, b, is the sum of the number of days lead
time multiplied by the probability of each lead time.

$b = (1 \times .25) + (2 \times .5) + (3 \times .25)$
$= .25 + 1.0 + .75$
$= 2.0$

The expected demand during lead time follows:

$$D = u \ b$$
$$= 1.0 \times 2.0$$
$$= 2.0$$

It will be recalled that $R = D + B$ and hence we still must calculate B before we can set a value for R. The value of the buffer stock will obviously depend on the extent of the fluctuation in the demand during lead time. There are essentially two ways of estimating the size and effects this fluctuation by evaluating the possible range of values that demand during lead time can take given the actual probability distributions or, alternatively assuming that demand during lead time is normally distributed and to determine the range of values and associated probabilities. We shall start with the assumption of normality.

Approach 1: Normally Distributed Demand During Lead Time

Demand during lead time can be assumed to follow the Normal distribution. You will recall that this means (i.a.) that certain proportions of results lie within specified ranges from the mean. For example, 90% of observations lie within 1.64 standard deviations from the mean whereas 95% of observations lie within 1.96 standard deviations from the mean.

One approach to using the buffer stock method of solving the probabilistic inventory model relies on these facts about the normal distribution. If we set a reorder point equal to the average demand during lead time plus 1.96 times the standard deviation of the distribution of demand during lead time, we will be able to cope with the demand during lead time in 95% of situations. The buffer stock method then rests on the assumption that managers are prepared to tolerate a certain frequency of stockouts. If, for example, the manager is prepared to allow stockouts to occur during 10% of the lead times then the buffer stock can be set at a particular level. If, on the other hand, the manager wants stockouts to only occur during 5% of the lead times and the buffer stock will have to be set at a higher level. (The manager should also be concerned lest the buffer stock be too large, hence it is important to note whether demand during a large number of lead times falls well below the expected demand.)

Clearly the calculation of the variance and the actual distribution of demand can be calculated from historical data but, for simplicity, it is often assumed that the variance of the distribution of demand during lead time is equal to the mean (i.e. Demand during lead time is assumed to be normally distributed with mean D and variance D). Since the standard deviation is the square root of the variance, we can immediately assume that the standard deviation of the demand during lead time is D.

The buffer stock that should be set will depend on the frequency of stock out that can be tolerated but we have the general formula –

$$B = k\sqrt{D}$$
where $k = 1.96$ for a 5% frequency of stock out

and we now have the formula for the reorder point

$$R = D + k\sqrt{D}$$

Example 2.3

Assume the procurement costs for a certain item are $20 per order placed and carrying costs are $100 per unit of inventory held for a year. Assume also the same distributio of lead time and demand as given in example 2.2 average demand day is 1 unit and expected demand during lead time is 2 units (i.e. as shown in Table 2.2). What should be the inventory policy which leads to a frequency of stock outs of 5%.

Let us start by determining the order quantity using the deterministic formula:

$$Q = \sqrt{\frac{2C_1 A}{C_2}}$$

$$C_1 = 20$$

$$C_2 = 100$$

As average demand per day is 1 unit, the total annual demand is 365 units (7 day week). The optimum order quantity is therefore

$$Q = \sqrt{\frac{2C_1 A}{C_2}}$$

$$= \frac{2 \times 20 \times 365}{100}$$

$$= 146$$

$$= 12.083$$

Since a total of 365 units are demanded, 30.21 orders must be placed. If we round these figures we should recommend that 31 orders of 12 units be placed (rounding 30.2 up to ensure demand is met).

Now to determine the reorder point

$$R = D + k\sqrt{D}$$

$$= 2 + 1.96\sqrt{2} \quad (k = 1.96 \text{ for 5\% stock out})$$

$$= 2 + 1.96 \times 1.414$$

$$= 2 + 2.77$$

$$= 4.77 \quad \text{and this should be rounded up to 5 units}$$

With this reorder point and 31 orders per year, stock out will only occur once.

Approach 2:   Calculating Actual Demand During Lead Time

The alternative approach to determining the appropriate buffer stock and hence the optimum reorder point is to calculate the actual probabilities of various levels of demand during lead time. Using the probability distribution given in example 2.2, we shall determine the possible levels of demand during lead time.

We can start this procedure by determining the possible range of values for (actual) demand during lead time. Since the shortest lead time is one day and the lowest demand per day is zero, the lowest possible demand during lead time is zero. On the other hand, as the longest possible lead time is three days and the largest demand per day is three units, the largest possible demand during lead time is nine units (i.e. three units being demanded on each of three days).

Obviously, the probability of each level of demand between zero and nine (inclusive) will depend on both the lead time probability (or, when a given level of demand can arise with more than one lead time, lead time probabilities) and the probability of the relevant combinations of demand per day that yield that demand.

The calculation of the probability of a demand of nine units occurring in the simplest, a demand of nine units will occur if there is a three day lead time (probability .25) and there is a demand of three units on each of those days.

Let P_k = probability of demand during lead time of k units

P_9 = probability of demand during lead time of nine units

= probability that there is a three day lead time _and_ there is a demand for three units on the first day of the lead time _and_ there is a demand for three units on the second day _and_ there is a demand for three units on the third day.

= .25 x (.1 x .1 x .1) (according to the rules of probability "and means multiply", i.e. we are concerned with the probability of the intersection of these events)

= .00025

Calculation of P_8 is only slightly more complicated as a demand of eight units can occur in three possible ways. These calculations are summarised below.

Demand During Lead Time	Patterns that can lead to this demand	Probability
9	3 day lead time	.25x
	3 units demanded first day, second day & third day	.1x .1x .1 = .00025
8	3 day lead time, 3, 3, 2 3, 2, 3 2, 3, 3	.25x {(.1x.1x.2) + (.1x.2x.1) + (.2x.1x.1)} = .0015

Note how in the calculation of P_8 the multiplicative law of probability is used (we are concerned with probability of demand of three units on first day and on second day and on third day - i.e. the <u>intersection</u> of these events), as well as the additive law (either demand of three day one and two on day two and three on day three <u>or</u> two on day one and three on the other two days i.e. we are concerned with the union of all these events).

The calculation of other values of P_k is more complicated because the number of possible combinations of lead times and levels of demand escalates. Consider, for example calculating P_6. A demand of six units can occur if there is a lead time of either two <u>or</u> three days (and so we will be concerned with the union of those two sets of events). When there is a two day lead time a demand if six units will occur if there is a demand of three units on the first day <u>and</u> a demand of three units on the second day (and so we will be concerned with the intersection of a two day lead time and demand of three units on each of those days). Of course there are many possibilities of a demand of six units if there is a three day lead time, including any of three groups of events: demand of three units on two days and zero units on the third day; two units on each of the three days <u>or</u> a demand of one unit on one day, two units on a second day and three units on the third day. All of these combinations add to six units. As the order of the occurrence of these events is important (in the sense that each one occurs with a distinct probability and each leads to a total demand six units), we can use probability theory to calculate how many ways we can order 3, 2 and 1 units. Alternatively, by a process of elimination we can specify each of the ways a demand of six units could occur:

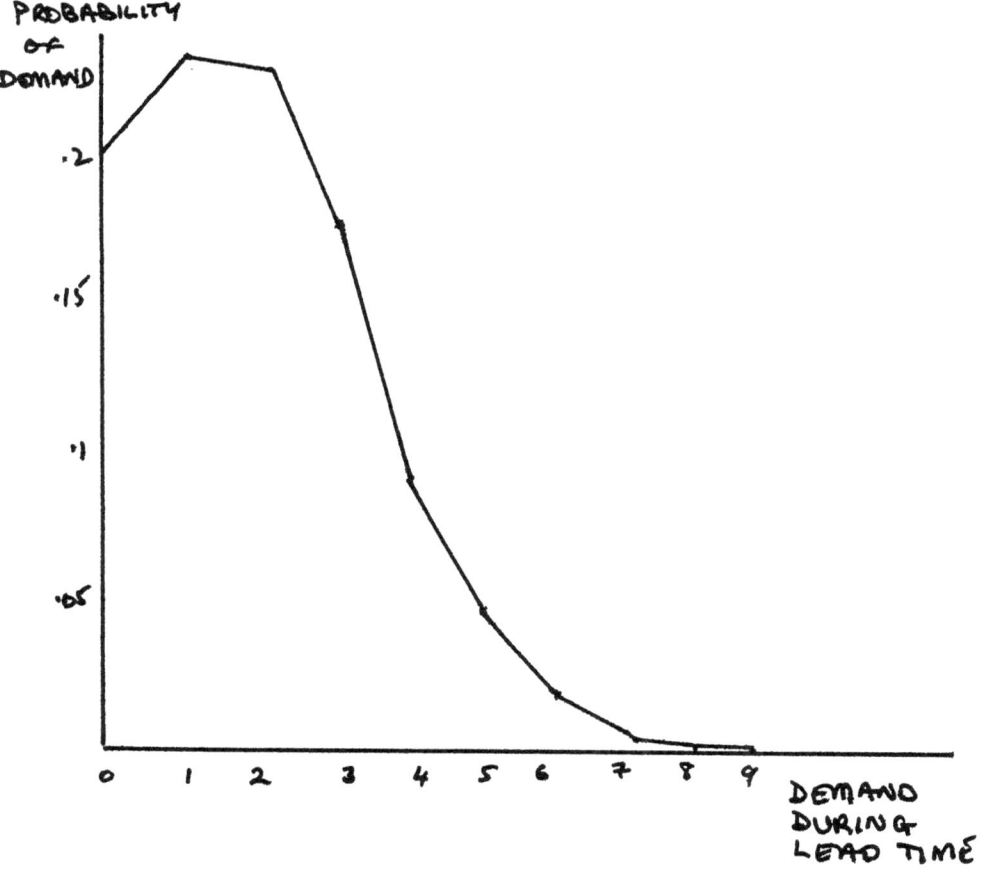

Figure 2.4

Clearly this figure is skewed to the left but it can be seen that most lead times are such that the demand during lead time is less than or equal to 2 units (the expected demand during lead time). With larger values of D, actual probabilities more closely approximate the normal distribution and hence support the use of approach 1 in determining the size of the buffer stock.

The example given is a simplification of the actual patterns which will face administrators, normally both lead time and demand will vary over a much wider range.

Tables of Values

Clearly any situation where stocks are held and order costs are significant can be examined for possible application of mathematical inventory models. In an attempt to reduce the highly mathematical orientation of the models the Oxford Regional Hospital Board has produced reports which include tables for calculating reorder quantity etc.

Unfortunately, the formulae given above may not provide completely realistic order quantities and so, to guard against order quantities which are either too large or too small, additional rules may be year's supply, the maximum order should

Demand During Lead Time	Patterns that can lead to this demand	Probability
6	3 day lead time,	.25x
	3, 3, 0	[(.1x.1x.4) +
	3, 0, 3	(.1x.4x.1) +
	0, 3, 3	(.4x.1x.1) +
	2, 2, 2	(.2z.2x.2) +
	3, 2, 1	(.1x.2x.3) +
	1, 2, 3	(.3x.2x.1) +
	1, 3, 2	(.3x.1x.2) +
	2, 1, 3	(.2x.3x.1) +
	2, 3, 1	(.2x.1x.3)]
	or 2 day lead time	+ .5 x (.1x.1)

$$\text{Thus } P_6 = .25 \ (.012 + .008 + .036) + .5 \text{ x } .01$$
$$= .014 + .005$$
$$= .019$$

Other values can be calculated similarly to yield Table 2.4.

Table 2.4

Demand During Lead Time	Probability of this demand
0	.1960
1	.2310
2	.2260
3	.1797
4	.0935
5	.0477
6	.0190
7	.0053
8	.0015
9	.0003
	1.0000

This table can be plotted

only be the annual consumption. If, however, the reorder quantity less than one month's supply, then the monthly consumption should be ordered. These rules have been systematised in published tables (e.g. see Oxford Regional Hospital Board, 1962).

Other tables relating acceptable average number of years between stockouts and order quantity have also been developed (Ammer, 1975: p.122). There are many computerised inventory packages available which, as well as providing billing and invoicing facilities, provide for calculation of reorder points and order quantities.

Mathematical model

The buffer stock model was one where the manager recognised that stockouts would occur and then specified a probability of stockouts that would be tolerable. No attempt was made to estimate the cost of the stockout and so, to that extent at least, the model does not take all variables into account. A mathematical model has been developed which involves estimating the cost of stockouts and is based on minimising the total inventory cost (including holding, ordering and stockout costs).

Let us define our symbols as before, together with a new term, C:

Q = Reorder quantity

A = Expected number of inventory items demanded per annum

C = Total Cost

C_1 = Procurement cost per order placed

C_2 = Carrying cost per unit of inventory held for the year

C_3 = Cost per unit out of stock

D = Expected demand during lead time.

Clearly our objective is to minimise the total inventory cost.

Now total cost,

   C = Procurement Cost + Holding Cost + Stockout Cost

Procurement cost will still obviously be the cost per order placed multiplied by the number of orders (as in the (deterministic model) i.e. $C_1 \frac{A}{Q}$

Carrying cost will similarly be related to that found in the deterministic model.

Figure 2.5 shows the limiting case where there is only one delivery per year.

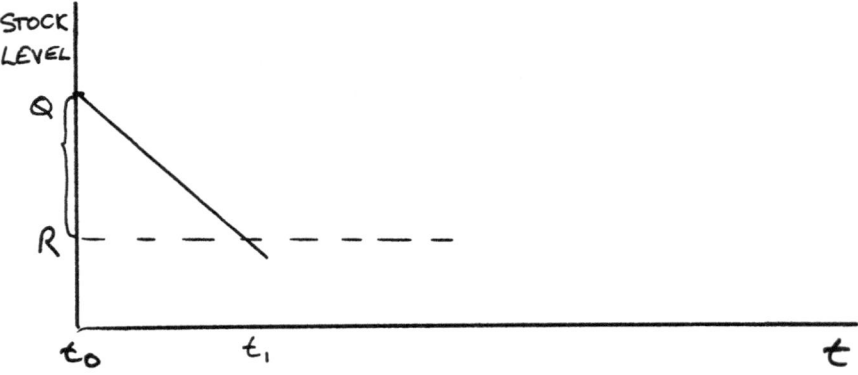

Figure 2.5

Clearly at t_0 (before the deliveries arrive) there are R - D units in stock (Reorder point - Demand since order placed). Hence when the orders are delivered there will be Q + (R - D) units in stock.

At the end of the period, t_1, there will still be R - D units in stock and hence the average number of units in stock will be

$$\frac{Q + (R - D) + R - D}{2}$$

$$= \frac{Q}{2} + R - D$$

It may be shown that this relationship holds true when demand, lead time and frequency of delivery are allowed to vary. Hence carrying cost will be $C_2 \left(\frac{Q}{2} + R - D\right)$.

As an aside it is interesting to note that in the deterministic model we effectively set R = D and our deterministic holding cost formula follows.

Stockout costs are now the only costs left to estimate. C_3, it will be recalled, is the cost per unit out of stock. Obviously the total annual cost for stockouts will depend on both the cost per unit out of stock and the number of units out of stock. In turn, the number of units out of stock will depend on the number of stockouts and their size. The size of the stockouts will vary according to the Reorder point. (The higher the reorder point, the lower will be both the size of stockout and its probability.) We shall now attempt to determine the expected size of stockouts.

Table 2.3 showed the relationships between different levels of demand during lead time and the probabilities of those levels. Using these figures let us consider the demand during lead time for a Reorder point of 9 units.

By definition a stockout occurs when the number of items in stock are insufficient to meet the demand. The expected value of a stockout will clearly be the size of the stockout multiplied by the probability of its' occurrence. Hence for a reorder point of 9:

$$\text{Expected size of stockout} = \text{(Excess number of units being demanded - number of units in stock) x probability of that number of units being demanded}$$

and since the greatest number of units that can be demanded is 9, the expected size of a stockout for a reorder point of 9 is zero. Now if we define $E(S_R)$ as the expected size of a stockout per lead time for reorder point R

$$E(S_9) = 0$$

Let us consider the case where the reorder point is 8 units. A stock out of size 1 can occur if there is a demand of 9 units during lead time. Such a demand will occur with a probability of .0003 (it will be recalled that we have calculated P_8, and indeed, other values of P_k earlier, see Table 2.4). The expected size of the stockout is thus 1 unit x .0003 = .0003.

The calculation of $E(S_6)$ is slightly more complicated:

$$\begin{aligned}
E(S_6) = \quad & \text{Expected size for demand of 9 units} \\
& +\text{Expected size for demand of 8 units} \\
& +\text{Expected size for demand of 7 units} \\
= \quad & \text{Size of Stockout x Prob. of Stockout for demand of 9 units} \\
& +\text{Size of Stockout x Prob. of Stockout for demand of 8 units} \\
& +\text{Size of Stockout x Prob. of Stockout for demand of 7 units} \\
= \quad & (9 - 6) \text{ x } .0003 +(8 - 6)\text{x } .0015 +(7 - 6)\text{x } .0053 \\
= \quad & 3 \text{ x } .0003 +2 \text{ x } .0015 +1 \text{ x } .0053 \\
= \quad & .0009 + .0030 + .0053 \\
= \quad & .0092
\end{aligned}$$

The method of calculation can be summarised as shown in Table 2.6.

Table 2.5

Reorder Point	Possible levels of Demand R	Resulting Stockout	Prob. of Demand	Expected size of this demand	$E(S_R)$
9	–	–	–	–	0
8	9	1	.0003	.0003	.0003
7	9	2	.0003	.0006	
	8	1	.0015	.0015	.0021
6	9	3	.0003	.0009	
	8	2	.0015	.0030	
	7	1	.0053	.0053	.0092

Similar values can be found for all other reorder points and they are shown in Table 2.6.

Table 2.6

Reorder Point R	Expected size of stockout per lead time for Reorder point R, ($E(S_R)$)
1	1.1864
2	0.6234
3	0.2764
4	0.1091
5	0.0353
6	0.0092
7	0.0021
8	0.0003
9	0.0000

Note that the reduction in the expected size of the stockout for a unit reduction in the reorder point is variable. For instance, if one reduces the order point from 9 to 8 units this would increase the expected size of stockouts per lead time by only .0003 units. If, on the other hand, we reduced the order point from 3 to 2 units, this would lead to an increase in the expected size of stockout of .347 units (.6234 − .2764). Thus at certain levels a significant reduction in holding costs may be achieved with practically no increase in stockout costs. In general, the attempt to make stockouts impossible in situations of probabilistic demand and lead time is almost certain to cost more than it is worth!

We now have sufficient information to calculate the cost associated with the expected annual stockouts.

Since C_3 = cost per unit out of stock

   $E(S_R)$ = expected size of stockout per lead time (for reorder point R)

   $C_3 \times E(S_R)$ = expected cost of stockout per lead time (for reorder point R).

By simply determining the number of lead times, we can then calculate the expected cost of all stockouts during the year.

When considering he deterministic model, we noted that if total demand is A units and the reorder quantity is Q units, the number of orders placed will be A/Q. But since lead time is defined as the delay between placement of an order and its' receipt, there must be the same number of lead times as orders placed, hence the number of lead times must also be A/Q. Thus the annual expected

stockout cost is $C_3 E(S_R)\dfrac{A}{Q}$.

Total cost can now be determined by summing the three component costs:

$$C = C_1 \frac{A}{Q} + C_2 \left(\frac{Q}{2} + R - D \right) + C_3 E(S_R) \frac{A}{Q}$$

It will be recalled that our objective is to determine values of R & Q such that C is minimised. Quite clearly the volume of calculations required to determine R & Q by trial and error ('iteration') is very large, but computer programs are available which will carry out the task in a few seconds. It should also be noted that for each reorder point there will be a specific order quantity which leads to a minimum cost and, at this order quantity any incremental change (whether up or down) will increase the cost. This fact can be used to reduce the number of calculations when it is necessary for them to be performed manually.

Example 2.4

Assume order costs are \$20, carrying costs are \$100 per unit held p.a. and stockout costs are \$40, with the probability distribution given in example 2.2, determine the optimum inventory policy.

Hence C_1 = 20

$\qquad C_2$ = 100

$\qquad C_3$ = 40

$\qquad A$ = 365

$\qquad D$ = 2

& Q & R are to be determined

Now as we are calculating a number of values we can rearrange our formula to group the two variables, Q & R, together:

$$C = C_1 \frac{A}{Q} + C_2 \left(\frac{Q}{2} + R - D\right) + C_3 \, E(S_R) \frac{A}{Q}$$

$$= C_1 \frac{A}{Q} + \frac{C_2}{2} (Q + 2R) - C_2 D + E(S_R) C_3 \frac{A}{Q}$$

$$= \frac{20 \times 365}{Q} + 50 (Q + 2R) - 100 \times 2 + E(S_R) \frac{40 \times 365}{Q}$$

$$= \frac{7300}{Q} + 50 (Q + 2R) - 200 + E(S_R) \frac{\times 14600}{Q}$$

For each of the different values of R and Q we can calculate C and hence, by iteration, find the combination of R and Q which yields the minimum cost (C).

For instance, if R = 3, Q = 10

$$C = \frac{7300}{10} + 50(10 + 6) - 200 + \frac{.2764}{10} \times 14600 \quad (E(S_R) \text{ is}$$

$$\text{taken from Table 2.7)}$$

$$= 730 + 800 - 200 + 403.55$$

$$= 1733.55$$

Table 2.7 shows the values of C for several different combinations of R and Q.

Table 2.7

	$\dfrac{7300}{Q}$	50(Q+2R)	$\dfrac{E(S_R) \times}{Q}$ 14600	$\dfrac{7300}{Q}$ + 50(Q+2R) + $\dfrac{E(S_R) \times 14600}{Q}$ − 200
R = 3				
Q = 10	730	800	403.555	1733.55
Q = 11	663.64	850	366.86	1680.50
Q = 12	608.33	900	336.29	1644.62
Q = 13	561.54	950	310.42	1621.96
Q = 14	521.43	1000	288.25	1609.68
Q = 15	486.67	1050	269.03	1605.70
Q = 16	456.25	1100	252.21	1608.46

Hence for R = 3, Q = 15 yields the minimum cost.

R = 4				
Q = 10	730	900	159.29	1589.29
Q = 11	663.64	950	144.81	1558.45
Q = 12	608.33	1000	132.74	1541.07
Q = 13	561.54	1050	122.53	1534.07
Q = 14	521.43	1100	113.77	1535.20

Hence for R = 4, Q = 13 yields the minimum cost.

R = 5				
Q = 10	730	1000	51.54	1581.54
Q = 11	663.64	1050	46.85	1560.49
Q = 12	608.33	1100	42.95	1551.28
Q = 13	561.54	1150	39.64	1551.18
Q = 14	521.54	1200	36.81	1558.24

Hence for R = 5, Q = 13 yields the minimum cost.

It can quickly be seen that a reorder point of 2 will be more expensive than one of 3 and similarly a reorder point of 6 will be more expensive than one of 5.

Hence the optimum inventory policy to pursue would be to place an order for 13 units whenever the level of inventory reaches 4 units. If this inventory policy is pursued, one can expect a stockout in 7.38% of lead times. (Since a demand of greater than 4 units will occur with probability of .0477 + .0190 + .0053 + .0015 + .0003 = .0738. Since there will be A/Q lead times (i.e. 365/13 = 28), we would expect approximately 2 stock outs per annum (7.38% of 28).

Conclusions concerning Mathematical Models

There are two significant conclusions concerning both probabilistic and deterministic models.

(a) The appropriate order quantity does not vary directly with demand.

Many hospitals and other institutions pursue inventory policies based on, say, holding one month's demand. It can quickly be seen that the higher the annual demand, the lower is the optimum average size of inventory per unit of demand. Hence if demand is 1,000 units and the optimum reorder point is 10 units this does not imply that when demand reaches 2,000 units the reorder point will be 20 units. In fact, a large number of other factors must be taken into account.

(b) The total cost of an optimum inventory is relatively insensitive to changes in most variables.

It is often argued that optimal inventory policies should not be developed because of the difficulties of measuring, say, stockout costs. But, because of the very nature of the model which takes into account other factors, the effect of an incorrect estimate of stockout cost is minimised.

Example 2.5

Using the data given in example 6.4 what would be the total inventory cost if stockout cost was increased from \$40 to \$60.

For a reorder point of 4 and an order quantity of 13, we previously found that total inventory cost would be \$1534.07 per annum. With the new stockout cost (50% increase), the total inventory cost is now

$$\frac{C_1 A}{Q} + \frac{C_2(Q + 2R)}{2} - C_2 D + \frac{E(S_R)C_3 A}{Q}$$

$$= 561.54 + 850 + \frac{.1091}{13} \times 60 \times 365$$

$$= 561.54 + 850 + 183.19$$

$$= 1595.33$$

i.e. the total inventory cost is now \$1595.33 which is a 3.9% increase. This procedure is known as 'sensitivity testing' and is discussed in more detail in Warner and Holloway (1978, pp.65-67).

APPLICATION OF INVENTORY THEORY

Many different types of problems can be viewed as inventory problems, some more realistically than others. Information is usually available in historical records concerning lead time distribution, distribution of demand etc. Of course, in some situations it is just not worth the effort of calculating optimum order policies for the myriad of goods held in a hospital store but it does seem reasonable that an inventory model should be developed for expensive items and those with a significant use.

It has been shown (Welch, 1965) that following a study of certain supply items:

A) 60% of total dollar investment was attributable to only 10% of the items
B) 35% of the investment was attributable to 35% of the items
C) 5% of the investment to 55% of the items

This is clear by applying inventory policies to only 10% of the items, significant savings on inventory costs could be made.

Ammer (1975, pp.106-113) discusses in some detail "A-B-C" analysis - techniques for inventory management of the three groups of items identified above.

Despite the fact that inventory theory could lead to clear improvement in the management of hospitals, it is not widely used. A survey of US hospitals by Ammer (1974) revealed that in 1973 most hospitals had essentially manual systems of inventory recording, although the preportion with computerised system increased with hospital size and over half of the larger hospitals used in-house computers for this purpose. The proportion of computer based inventory system in use has probably increased dramatically since then.

The conclusions of a survey of the use of inventory theory in British companies are also pertinent (Muhlemann & Lockett, 1978, p.230).

"The most conclusive result was that larger companies tended, naturally enough, to have more sophisticated systems. Whether more sophisticated systems result in 'better' control of inventory is another matter. There is a real difficulty in measuring the 'goodness' of inventory systems against each other, designers are prone to claim muilitudes of intangible unquantifiable benefits...

There did appear to be some evidence that some organisations were using quite sophisticated formal models of inventory control... These tended to be the larger organisations where 'scientific management' had already gained a substantial foothold, and hence management had been educated to accepted this approach. In those smaller organisations with sophisticated systems, there tended to be a person in a key position responsible for the system, with the personality, drive, enthusiasm, ability to convince others to accept the system, and work with it. Moreover there was evidence that those companies with sophisticated systems felt they were ahead of competitors, and were therefore reluctant to discuss their models in any real depth."

Importantly, it is possible to develop measures of performance of inventory systems and compare hospitals on variables such as purchasing prices; cost of materials per bed, acquisition and cost of purchasing per dollar of purchases (see Ammer, 1974; p.119). Use of such comparisons may encourage hospitals to improve efficiency in this area.

One reason why inventory policies are not adopted in hospitals is the difficulty in quantifying stockout costs, notwithstanding the fact that many types of stockout costs can easily be calculated. Stockout costs can be usefully classified as follows:

1) Direct costs associated with expediting orders or providing substitutes for the particular item demanded.

2) Indirect costs involved in revenue lost by not being able to provide the service for which the item is required.

3) Humanitarian costs associated with patient discomfort, pain and, in extreme circumstances, death.

4) Institutional costs associated with the morale of staff and patients or the hospital's image in the community.

It should be recalled, however, that an optimum inventory policy always exists. Unfortunately, inventory policies as currently exist are based on the assumption that the hospital should never run out of any item be it cornflakes, cotton balls or blood. But this necessarily means that the administrator is imputing a cost (possible infinite) to stockouts even though the community does not value human pain, discomfort or life infinitely.

As you recall the formula for the probabilistic inventory model is:

$$ C = C_1 \frac{A}{Q} + C_2 (\frac{Q}{2} + R - D) + C_3 E(S_R) \frac{A}{Q} $$

A typical hospital inventory policy is at best expressed as "if there are only 100 boxes left put an order in for another 1000 boxes". Such a policy places a value on R & Q, and because lead times are externally determined and demand can be estimated from historical data, values for $E(S_R)$, D & A follow. Accounting data can provide information on total costs of inventory policies, ordering costs and carrying costs, hence C, C_1 and C_2 can be quantified. Thus the only value not yet quantified is C_3, the stockout cost, and the equation could be solved to find a value for C_3. Despite the protestations of many, hospitals can be seen to be implicitly evaluating stockout costs.

As the optimal policy involves a balance between procurement costs, carrying costs and stockout costs, any attempt to ensure that stockouts are impossible (i.e. placing an infinite value on stockout costs) necessarily implies that either frequent ordering or high levels of inventories are necessary. These policies would probably in the long run cause a greater cost than allowing occasional stockouts.

Hospital Stores

Smith et al have reported a series of operations research studies relating to inventory and stores control in hospitals in the United Kingdom (Smith, Gregory & Maguire, 1975). These studies commenced in 1969 and involved the development of easily used tables for inventory control. Although optimum inventory policies (such as the mathematical formulation discussed above) involve simultaneously determining order quantity and reorder point, the U.K. studies opted for sub-optimisation in the interests of ease of implementation and separate rules for order quantity and reorder point were developed.

Following investigation, order costs were assumed to be £0.25 per item per order. (Note order costs here vary with the size of the order.) Although the research team made a number of estimates of carrying costs, the final tables they developed did not involve a specific value for these but rather relied on different rules for bulky (>½ cubic foot per pound sterling) and non bulky items. An order quantity table was derived and published (Table 2.8).

Table 2.8 Derived Order Quantity Table

Annual Turnover (£) items < ½ cu. ft/£	Order Quantity (week's supply)	Annual Turnover (£) items > ½ cu. ft/£
Less than £10		Less than £4
10 - 40£		4 - 15£
40 - 160 £		15 - 60£
160 - 650£		60 - 250£
650 - 2,600£		250 - 1,000£
More than 2,600£		More than 1,000£

The team involved in the inventory project also analysed patterns of demand for a number of items and found it to be constant! The distribution of lead time was studied and found to follow a negative exponential distribution and thus patterns for demand during lead time established.

"Service Levels" (defined as the "proportion of orders made by the store that arrive before the stock runs out" p.379) were derived for major groups of items and a simplified reorder level table produced (Table 2.9).

Table 2.9 Derived Reorder Level Table

Re-order level = longest lead-time (weeks) over last ten orders x average weekly demand x safety factor

Commodity Class	Service Levels	Safety Factor
Groceries, bedding and linen, building and engineering, stationery, furniture and fittings fittings.	95.0%	1.00
Hardware and crockery, cleaning materials, staff uniforms; patients' clothing, sewing room sundries	97.5%	1.25
Medical and surgical equipment, (including instruments), dressings.	99.0%	1.50

The inventory policy system described in the Smith et al paper has been implemented in the U.K. A similar paper, drawing heavily on the U.K. work has been developed by the New Zealand Department of Health (Smith & Moir, 1979).

Blood Banks

The application of inventory models to blood banks has attracted considerable attention (viz. Stimson & Stimson, 1972, pp.21-23; Fries, 1981, pp.68-72. The blood bank has clear holding costs since blood held for a certain length of time cannot be used and order costs can easily be measured. In one study (Silver & Silver, 1964), measurements of 'expiration costs' were made and an inventory model formulated. It was noted that "Emergency usage' of the blood costs more than normal usage and discussed different methods of assessing 'expediting costs'. The following table of costs were found to occur.

Table 2.10   Blood Storage Costs

Stock Level	Expirations over 18 month period	Expirations as % of total usage	Cost at $15 per expirat- ions	No. of Expediting Situations	Expediting cost	Total cost
9-13	0	0	0	17	510	510
14-18	15	1.6	300	7	210	543
19-23	75	8.0	1125	3	90	1215
24-28	165	17.6	2425	0	0	2475

The new system was implemented and total costs were reduced with a simultaneous reduction in expediting costs and the provision of fresher blood to patients. As this study was undertaken in the United States where there is a market price for blood, measurement of holding costs was simplified. However it is interesting to note the use of 'expediting costs' as a measure of stock-out costs.

Mergers and Centralisation

Reinke (1972, p.258) has used inventory models to quantify the issues surrounding mergers of hospital facilities. He suggests that the total capacity of a hospital should be the average usage plus three times the square root of the usage.

An analysis of a related area, the benefits of centralisation, was undertaken by Smith, Gregory and Maguire (1975). They analysed the costs associated with different warehousing policies, the results of which are summarised in Table 2.11.

Table 2.11 Comparison of 1971 Costs for Three Different Stores
            Options

		Hospital Stores	Area Warehouse plus sub-stores at hospitals	Area Central Stores
Supplies Cost	(£ p.a.)	450,000	450,000	450,000
Manpower Costs	(£ p.a.)	70,100	72,400	29,300
Operating Costs	(£ p.a.)	24,600	18,300	16,700
Transport Costs	(£ p.a.)	–	3,000	3,000
Totals	(£ p.a.)	94,700	93,700	49,000

It can be seen that the theoretically predicted advantages were
found in practice.

Training Programs

Inventory models can also be applied to staffing situations.
Grundy and Reinke (1973, p.48) discuss the following situation:

"A programme administrator requires the services of 48
laboratory technicians; since they remain for only two years
on the average, he must recruit and train a new batch of
candidates at intervals. Frequent training courses are
costly, but are necessary if there is not to be unavoidable
over-staffing at times to allow for attrition during the
intervals between replacements. Should training courses be
conducted annually, semi annually or quarterly?"

Clearly this is a typical inventory problem. These are "carrying
costs" involved in keeping the trainees employed over the daily
work requirement and there are "order costs" involved in running
training courses. "Stock-outs" will have to be avoided by
training sufficient staff. Quantifications of the costs can be
made by looking at salary costs etc. and an optimal policy
calculated.

Conclusions

Many managers would probably endorse Gue and Freeman's (1975)
conclusions about the use of inventory theory:

"..the cost of conducting the requisite studies in the
hospital environment, where good usage data are scarce and
certain costs difficult to measure, is rarely justified by
the return. A hard-nosed and experienced purchasing agent, a
good stock-keeping system that is coupled with sufficient
foresight to avoid being caught with a large supply of
obsolescent items, and continuous attempts to standardize can
often save considerably more than scientifically derived
Economic Order Quantities and reorder points."

They are probably overly sceptical. However, there are significant limitations involved in the use of inventory models in the health care field.

It is useful, though, to understand the principles and assumptions underlying the mathematical model and the implications of the solution obtained. The models may then help to conceptualise many of the difficulties faced by managers. Even more importantly, computerised inventory packages are increasingly available, thus facilitating the use of quantified inventory models.

REFERENCES

Ammer, D.S. (1974) Hospital Materials Management: Neglect & Inefficiency Promote High Costs of Care, Bureau of Business & Economic Research, Northeastern University.

Ammer, D.S. (1975) Purchasing & Materials Management for Health Care Institutions, Lexington.

Fries, B.E. (1981) Applications of Operations Research to Health Care Delivery Systems: A Complete Review of the Periodical Literature, (Lecture Notes in Medical Informatics No. 10), Springer Verlag.

Grundy, F. & Reinke, W.A. (1973) Health Practice Research and Formalized Managerial Methods, (Public Health Papers No. 51), WHO.

Gue, R.L. & Freeman, J.R. (1975) "Information Systems" in Shuman, L.J., Speas, R.D. & Young, J.P. (eds.) Operations Research in Health Care: A Critical Analysis, Johns Hopkins University Press.

Muhlemann, A.P. & Lockett, A.G. (1978) 'The Use of Formal Inventory Control Models: A Preliminary Survey', Omega: The International Journal of Management Science, Vol. 6, No. 3, pp.227-230.

Oxford Regional Hospital Board, (1962) Optimum Purchasing Policy, (Operational Research Unit Report No. 4), Oxford.

Oxford Regional Hospital Board, (1962) Optimum Purchasing Tables, (Operational Research Unit Report No. 5), Oxford.

Reinke, W.A. (1972) Health Planning: Qualitative Aspects & Quantitative Techniques, Department of International Health, School of Hygiene & Public Health, John Hopkins University.

Silver, A. & Silver, A.M. (1964) 'An empirical inventory control system fo hospital blood banks', Hospitals J.A.H.A., 38 (Aug. 1) pp.56-72.

Smith, A.G., Gregory, K. & Maguire, J.D. (1975) 'Operational Research for the Hospital Supply Service', Operational Research Quarterly, Vol. 26, No. 2, ii pp.375-388.

Smith, A. & Moir, G. (1979) Hospital Stores - Stock Control & Guidelines on Accommodation, Management Services & Research Unit, Department of Health, Wellington.

Stimson, D.H. & Stimson, R.H. (1972) Operations Research in Hospitals, H.R.E.T.

Warner, D.M. & Holloway, D.C. (1978) Decision Making & Control for Health Administration: The Management of Quantitative Analysis, Health Administration Press.

Welch, W.E. (1957) Tested Scientific Inventory Control, Management Publishing Co.

INVENTORY SUMMARY

An inventory has been defined as a store of items standing idle awaiting use. The inventory problem is to determine the optimum number of items that should be held taking into account the costs associated with holding or not holding the inventory.

Three inventory models were outlined, all of which involve determining the reorder point and the optimum order quantity.

Definitions:

C = Total cost
C_1 = Procurement cost per order placed
C_2 = Carrying cost per unit of inventory held for year.
C_3 = Cost per stockout
A = Annual demand
Q = Reorder quantity
R = Reorder point
$E(S_R)$ = Expected size of stockout per lead time (for reorder point R)
D = Expected demand during lead time
B = Size of buffer stock

1) Deterministic model

* Reorder point determined by lead time
* Optimum Order quantity to be determined by formula:

$$Q = \sqrt{\frac{2C_1 A}{C_2}}$$

2) Buffer stock model

* Reorder point determined by demand during lead time plus a buffer stock to cope with random variation.

$$R = D + B$$

One can assume that demand during lead time is normally distributed with mean D and standard deviation D and it follows that

$R = D + k\sqrt{D}$ where k is a normal variate chosen to reflect the desired probability of stock out.

* Order quantity determined as in deterministic model.

3) Mathematical model

* Reorder point and order quantity chosen (by process of iteration) so that total cost of inventory is minimised.

$$C = C_1 \frac{A}{Q} + C_2 \left(\frac{Q}{2} + R - D\right) + C_3 E(S_R)\frac{A}{Q}$$

3   QUEUING

All administrators have been faced with problems concerning
waiting time.   Many of the complaints received by hospital
executives relate to alleged excessive waits in Radiology, the
Emergency Room etc.   Excessive waiting time is obviously bad for
the hospital: it can lead to both decline in the hospital's image
in its community as well as occasional medical mishaps.   We have
also all heard innumerable horror stories of hospital waiting
times: people waiting hours or alternatively, the place being so
deserted that the arriving patient does not dare wake the
sleeping staff.   These examples are all symptoms of problems in
the system.   Rising (1977, p3) describes the situation thus:

> "Hurry up and wait", frustration, long waiting times for
> patients, and the staff being alternately harassed and
> overworked, then idle, are symptoms of a poorly designed
> system for patient flow.   These symptoms occur in many
> different types of outpatient facilities including medical
> clinics, group practices, emergency rooms, and large hospital
> outpatient departments.   There are even patient flow problems
> in the offices of solo practitioners.
>
> Patients who are late for appointments, "no-shows,"
> emergencies that disrupt schedules, and "lost" records and
> specimens are typical of the reasons given for the delays.
> However, these immediate reasons are not the cause of the
> problem; the real reason for the problem is that the basic
> principles of systems analysis and design were not
> considered when the facility was designed.   The confusion in
> poorly designed systems makes it easy to "lose" things; each
> emergency becomes a crisis instead of an occasion to
> implement a contingency plan, and late patients and "no-
> shows" cause physicians to be idle while they wait for the
> next patient.

Often managers claim that patient demand can't be predicted; that
"you can't control the docs" or that the incident was an
abberation.   These are all essentially excuses for bad management
or poor systems.   Queuing theory has been developed to assist
managers to analyse problems of queues or waiting-lines and to
develop improved systems.   Queuing problems occur commonly and
generalised solutions have been developed.

Queuing theory assumes the existence of a facility at which work
is done or a service performed and where customers arrive,
requiring service.

The "customer" may be letters requiring a signature, cars to be
packed, ships to be unloaded, parts to be assembled, or people
requiring attention in a bank, a cafeteria or in a hospital

outpatient department. The waiting customers form a queue or a waiting line. The whole operation of the system is referred to as the queuing process.

The common operations research balancing situation exists. On the one hand, if customers arrive too frequently they will have to wait for the service (or do without it). On the other hand, if they arrive too infrequently the service facilities will remain idle between arrivals.

In general there will be costs associated with providing a service and, of course, with any idle time associated with the service. There will also be costs associated with the waiting time which customers spend in the queue (or with customers doing without the service if the queue is too long). Phrased another way, there will be costs associated with providing a certain level of service and there will be costs associated with providing only that level of service.

Clearly, the more or the larger the service facilities provided, the smaller will be the queues which tend to form and hence the smaller will be the costs which are associated with waiting. On the other hand, the greater the capacity of the service facilities, the greater will be the costs of providing the service and the greater will be the tendency for the service to be idle on some occasions, with a consequent increase in costs from this source.

The objective in dealing with queuing problems is to provide a level of facilities, or otherwise influence the queuing process, so that the overall costs associated with the process are minimized.

Jones (1972) describes the situation as follows:

"The problem with queuing situations is simply this. Arrival is not generally regular... We can do a survey and calaculate average arrival rates at different times of the day and do all sorts of analysis, but we can never predict exactly when the next customer will arrive... Similarly, service times may vary, particularly if the service involves a human element, and is not fully automated.

So sometimes arrivals occur in bursts, so that a queue inevitably forms, while at other times, because of a long gap between arrivals, the service facilities will be idle. The variation in service times adds further complication in that at times the queue will be faster moving than at other times. This all means that there is no simple relationship between the service facilities provided and the demand for service. So even if we provide service facilities which have more capacity than the demand, we may still have queues forming.

In a nutshell, the economics of the situation are that we provide a service which clearly has a cost associated with it, and against this we have the cost of losing custom or delaying our production if queues form. It is the ideal balance between these costs that we seek, bearing in mind of course our policy with respect to the level of service we wish to offer. (We may wish to avoid queues at all costs if we operate a Bond Street hairdressing salon, but the cost of our service will be proportionally high.)

ELEMENTS OF QUEUING PROBLEMS

Queuing theory has been developed in an attempt to solve these problems. The many different queuing problems have certain common elements, and nine elements of any problem can be identified:

(1) There is a facility providing a service

The 'facility' may be the emergency room or obstetric suite of a hospital, or the pay office. Each facility will be different but the problems of all are the same.

(2) There are customers who arrive to use this facility

The customers may be either patients seeking treatment or staff waiting for their pay.

(3) Within the facility there are servers who provide service to the customers

In the emergency room, there would be one or more medical practitioners who treat the patients; in the obstetric suite the servers could probably best be characterised as the beds; in the pay office, the server would be the pay officers. It is important to note that each facility can have any number of servers.

(4) The customers arrive in a certain pattern and at a certain rate

Typically customers will arrive at the unit in a certain way. It may be random, it may depend on the bus timetable, it may be perfectly predictable but there is almost invariably some pattern. Common arrival patterns are:

(a)   Constant or deterministic arrival pattern (arrows
        denoting arrivals).

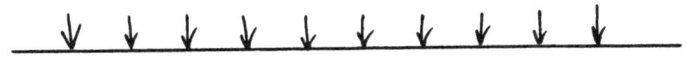

(b)   Variable arrival pattern.

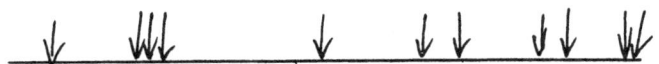

(c)   Bunched arrival pattern (constant).

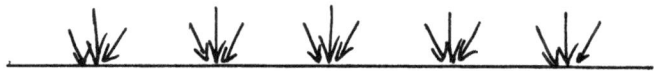

Figure 3.1

To specify completely the nature of the arrival process, we
must know not only the arrival pattern, but also the arrival
rate. Thus, for example, a constant or deterministic arrival
pattern could have people arriving every two minutes or every
five minutes. Although the pattern is the same in both cases,
the arrival rate is different.

The arrival rate may be defined as the number of customers who
arrive at the facility seeking service per unit of time. Where
arrivals follow a probability distribution, the arrival rate is
to be interpreted as the mean of the probability distribution
i.e. the expected number of arrivals per unit of time.   It
should be remembered in those cases that the value of the
arrival rate is an average; actual arrival could be bunched or
spread out in an irregular manner.

Administrators often claim that arrivals at an emergency unit,
for example, are completely random: this is often not the case
as they are affected by bus timetables, traffic lights etc.
Despite this, most mathematical queuing models assume that
arrivals are random.   Randomness in mathematical terms has a
very strict meaning (there is nothing random about 'random'!).

Random arrivals have two main attributes.   First, they are
homogeneous i.e. the probability of an event occurring in any
small unit of time is constant, on the average.   In queuing
problems this is interpreted to mean that the arrival rate is
constant over the period being examined. Thus emergency room
managers expect more attendances on Monday mornings than on
Tuesday mornings, arrivals between 2 am and 3 am are not
as frequent as arrivals between 10 pm and 11 pm. However, the

arrival rate can be assumed to be constant within each (homogeneous) period.

Secondly, events (or arrivals) in any one time interval are independent of events (or arrivals) in that or any other time interval. Thus if there has been one arrival in time interval 3, this does not affect the probability of there being one arrival in time interval 4. As Hollingdale (1978) concludes:

"A random sequence of arrivals is in fact a very special pattern of arrivals; there is nothing vague about it notwithstanding the popular connotation of the word 'random'. It is a good approximation to reality when the customers are drawn from a large group who all behave independently. Another of its attractions is that it is easy to handle mathematically!"

Poisson Arrivals.

It can be shown (see, for instance, Wagner 1969:843) that there is a mathematical distribution which can be used to approximate random arrivals. This distribution is known as the <u>Poisson distribution</u>, and events which are distributed randomly over a period of time are said to follow the Poisson distribution. The distribution is named after the French mathematician, S.D. Poisson (1781-1840).

Given the assumptions of randomness described above, the probability of r arrivals in a period of time, T, simply depends on the value of the average arrival rate and the length of the time interval T.

The Poisson distribution can be defined in terms of the probability of a given number of arrivals (r) in any unit of time as follows:

$$P \text{ (r arrivals in unit of time)} = \frac{e^{-\lambda}\lambda^r}{r!}$$

where e is a very famous mathematical constant, the base of natural logarithms

$e = 2.71828$
λ = arrival rate per unit of time
$r! = r \times (r-1) \times (r-2) \times (r-3) \times \ldots . 3 \times 2 \times 1$

Clearly the probability of a given number of arrivals varies with the arrival rate. For example, if there are, on average, 2 arrivals every minute, =2. The probability of there being 0,1,2,3,....arrivals in any minute can be derived from the formula:

$$P\text{(r arrivals in any unit of time)} = \frac{e^{-\lambda}\lambda^r}{r!}$$

$$P\text{(0 arrivals in any unit of time,} = \frac{e^{-2}2^0}{0!} \text{ (since } \lambda = 2; \ r = 0).$$
in this case a minute)

$$= \frac{1}{e^2}$$

$$= .1353 \text{ (using tables, logarithms or calculators)}$$

Similarly, $P(1 \text{ arrival in a minute}) = \dfrac{e^{-2}2^1}{1!}$

$$= .1353 \times 2$$

$$= .2706$$

$P(2 \text{ arrivals in a minute}) = \dfrac{e^{-2}2^2}{2!}$

$$= \dfrac{.1353 \times 4}{2}$$

$$= .1353 \times 2$$

$$= .2706$$

$P(3 \text{ arrivals in a minute}) = \dfrac{e^{-2}2^3}{3!}$

$$= \dfrac{.1353 \times 8}{6}$$

$$= .1804$$

Other values can be calculated in a similar manner.

Figure 3.2 shows the shape of the Poisson distribution for $\lambda = 2$. The values shown in this curve are derived from the calculations above.

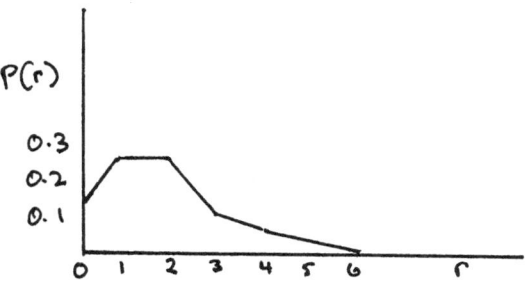

Figure 3.2

The shape of the Poisson distribution varies with λ. Figure 3.3 shows the shape of the Poisson curve for different values of λ, the arrival rate.

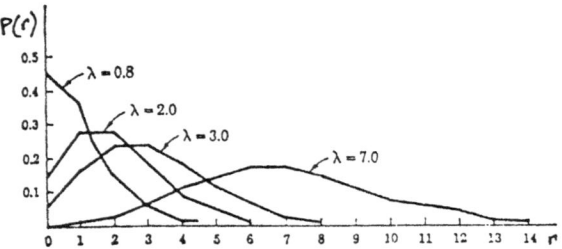

Figure 3.3

Rather than specifying the arrival pattern in terms of a
probability distribution of the probabilities of r arrivals in a
unit of time, some operations research studies specify the
arrival pattern in terms of the probability distribution of the
times between arrivals - sometimes called 'inter-arrival times'.
It can be shown that the Poisson arrival pattern implies that
interarrival times are distributed according to the negative
exponential distribution.

(5) **The servers are arranged in a particular way**

Emergency rooms are often arranged so that patients can see any
one of a number of medical practitioners. This type of
arrangement is known as a situation where servers are 'in
parallel'. Once a patient has seen the doctor he or she may have
to go to radiology, where another wait in a queue may be
involved. When a patient has to see one server and then another,
the arrangement of servers is said to be 'in series' or
'multiphase'.

Many different arrangements can exist, some of which are shown in
Figure 3.4

QUEUING SYSTEMS

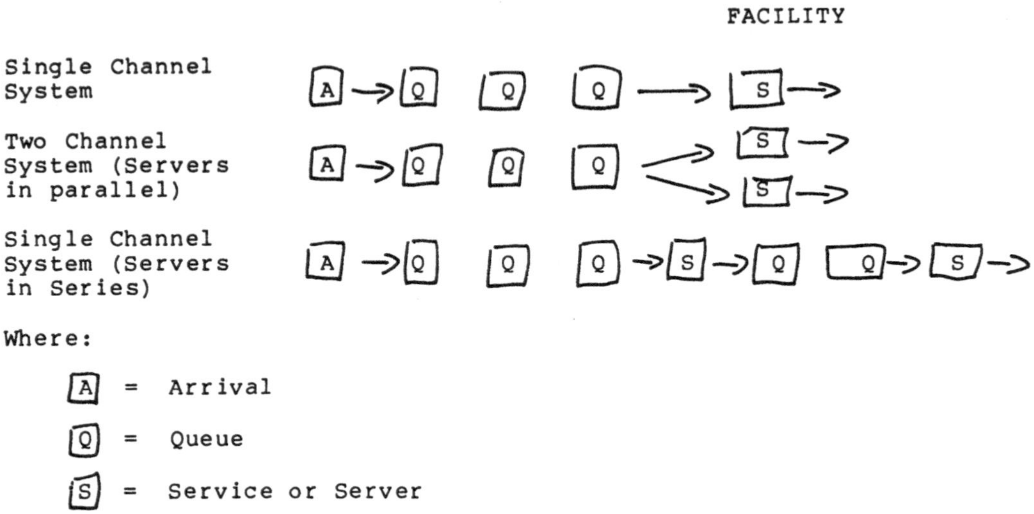

                                                    FACILITY

Single Channel
System   A → Q   Q   Q ⟶ S →

Two Channel
System (Servers   A → Q   Q   Q ⟹ S →
in parallel)   ⟹ S →

Single Channel
System (Servers   A → Q   Q   Q → S → Q   Q → S →
in Series)

Where:

    A = Arrival

    Q = Queue

    S = Service or Server

Figure 3.4

(6) <u>The customers are served in a particular order</u>

All queuing systems involve some rules concerning the order in which customers are served and these describe the <u>queue discipline</u>. In a hospital situation two major rules are normally followed.

(a) 'First come, first served'.
     This is common in radiology departments, pay offices, general-practice type departments etc.

(b) Emergencies first.
     This is common naturally enough, in emergency type departments.

The two types of rules can, of course, be operated in the same facility where, for instance, emergencies are seen first and others seen on a 'first come, first served' basis. A rule which may also be used is to give preference to patients whose service time is likely to be low although the use of this rule is not widespread.

(7) <u>The customers are served in a certain pattern and at a certain rate</u>

Just as customers arrive in a certain pattern, there are patterns which describe their treatment times, called, naturally enough, the <u>service pattern</u>. All customers may, for example, only take five minutes to be seen and treated; on the other hand, some may take longer than others. The simplest service pattern is the deterministic one i.e. all patients are seen for exactly the same length of time and the system is strictly determined (this situation parallels the deterministic arrival pattern where patients arrive at given time intervals). An assumption of a deterministic service pattern is usually unrealistic and in most situations, a probability distribution provides a more accurate representation of the service pattern. One can debate what is the most appropriate probability distribution to use and this will obviously vary from case to case, however, the most commonly used service distribution is the <u>negative exponential</u> pattern.

The negative exponential distribution reflects the situation where most patients only require short consultations while a small number of patients require long consultations.

Just as there is an arrival pattern and an arrival rate, so too there is a service pattern and a <u>service rate</u>. The service rate is defined as the output of the service facility per time unit that the facility is in operation. (Note that this definition implies that the service rate does not include time during which the facility is not operating.)

The inverse of the service rate is the <u>mean service time</u> or the average time for each unit of output.

An elementary proof:

$$\text{Service rate} = \frac{\text{Output}}{\text{time unit}}$$

$$= \frac{1}{\dfrac{\text{time unit}}{\text{output}}}$$

$$= \frac{1}{\text{mean service time}}$$

When a probability distribution applies it is appropriate to use the expected service rate which is commonly denoted μ (mu).

The formula for the negative exponential distribution is

$$y = \mu e^{-\mu t}$$

where y = frequency of given service time
μ = service rate
t = time

This formula can be used in two ways. First and most simply is to plot the frequency (or relative frequency) of the occurrence of given service times.

Example 3.1

Let us consider the situation where the average service time is 15 minutes (hence 4 persons are seen per hour and μ = 4) and the service times are distributed negative exponentially.

Now $y = \mu e^{-\mu t}$

$$= 4e^{-4t}$$

Let us first examine the frequency of a service time of 10 minutes (1/6 hour = 0.166).

$$y = 4e^{-4t}$$

$$= 4e^{-4 \times 0.166} \text{ (substituting t = 0.166)}$$

$$= 4e^{-0.666}$$

$$= 4 \times .5151 \text{ (from tables)}$$

$$= 2.06$$

Thus a service time of 10 minutes is expected to occur about twice.

A service time of 15 minutes ($\frac{1}{4}$ hour; t = .25) will occur:

$$y = 4e^{-4 \times 0.25}$$

$$= 4e^{-1}$$

$$= 4 \times .36788$$

$$= 1.47 \text{ times}$$

A service time of 20 minutes (.33 hours) will occur:

$$y = 4e^{4 \times 0.33}$$

$$= 4e^{-1.333}$$

$$= 4 \times .2636$$

$$= 1.05 \text{ times}$$

The following table summarises the distribution:

Service time (Minutes)	Frequency
5	2.87
10	2.06
15	1.47
20	1.05
30	.54
45	.19
60	.07

This can be represented graphically:

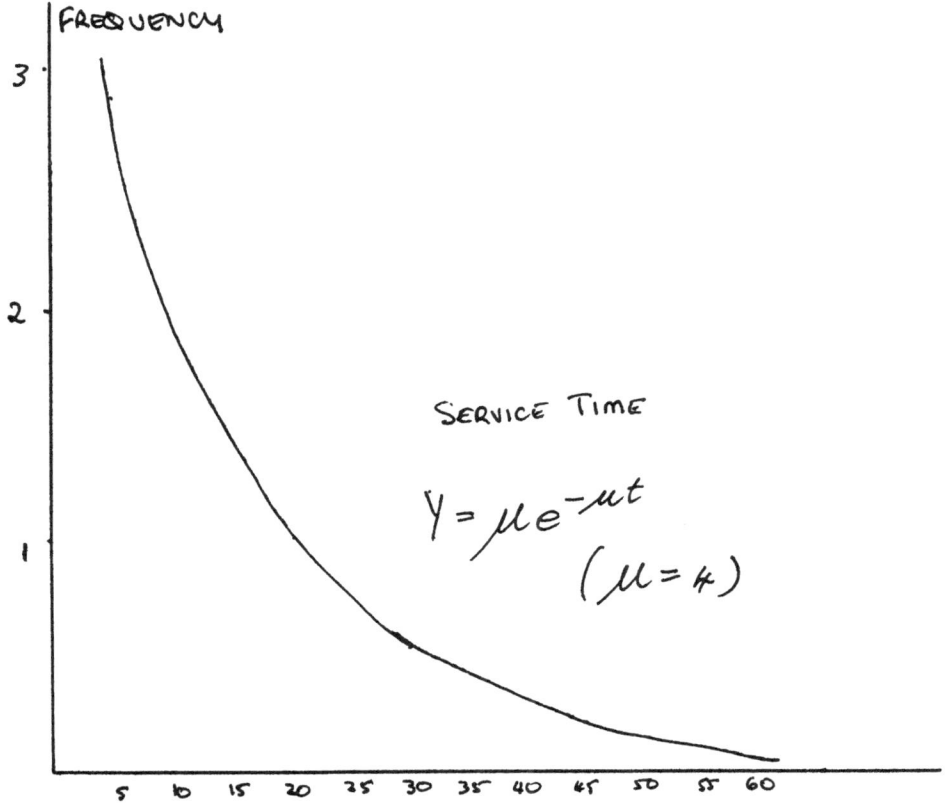

Figure 3.5

It can be quickly seen that the negative exponential distribution indeed reflects the situation where a large number of patients require a short consultation but a small number of patients require a long consultation.

The second way in which the service time formula can be used is to derive expected values for use in testing goodness of fit using the chi-square distribution. Let us assume, for example, that we undertook a survey of an outpatient department which has a service rate of four per hour. In this survey we recorded service time to the nearest five minutes and we saw 100 patients who had service time of between 5 minutes and two hours (the results of the survey are not shown here.)

We could use the formula $y = e^{-t}$ to calculate a frequency distribution for each of the possible values (Table 3.1, column 2); sum this (Table 3.1, sum of column 2 - 10.109) and use this to calculate an expected frequency for the situation where there are 100 people served (Table 3.1, column 2 - 10.109 x 100). If the conditions for using chi-square apply we could then test our survey data to see whether the negative exponential distribution provides a reasonable representation of reality.

Table 3.1 Frequency Distribution for Service Times

Service Time (Minutes)	Relative Frequency	Expected Values
Column (1)	Column (2)	Column (3)
5	2.8662	28.35
10	2.0538	20.32
15	1.4717	14.56
20	1.0545	10.43
25	.7556	7.47
30	.5414	5.36
35	.3880	3.84
40	.2780	2.75
45	.1992	1.97
50	.1427	1.41
55	.1023	1.01
60	.0723	.73
65	.0525	.52
70	.0376	.37
75	.0270	.27
80	.0193	.19
85	.0138	.14
90	.0099	.10
95	.0071	.07
100	.0051	.05
105	.0037	.04
110	.0026	.03
115	.0019	.02
120	.0013	.01
TOTAL	10.109	100.0

Of course, service times are not always best portrayed by the negative exponential distribution. Another distribution that is occasionally used in queuing studies is the Gamma distribution. The formula for the distribution is as follows:

$$g(y) = \frac{a(ay)^{b-1}e^{-ay}}{(b-1)!}$$

Where g(y) = frequency of service times of y and the mean   of the distribution is b/a.

The Gamma distribution is related to the Erlang distribution and in fact replacing 'a' by 'an' in the formula above, yields the formula for the Erlang distribution of order nx. Figure 3.5 shows the shape of the Gamma distribution for a=1 and b=1; b=3; b=6; and b=10.

The Gamma Distribution

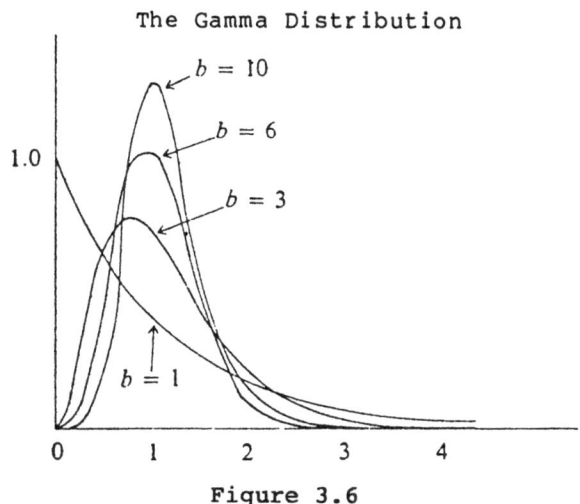

Figure 3.6

(8)   There is a cost to the customer (Positive or negative) caused by being at the facility

(9)   There is a cost to the community caused by the existence of the facility (This is sometimes known as the service cost)

Luck et al (1971) comments on these further elements of queuing systems as follows:

"In queueing problems in an industrial context it is often quite easy to get explicit money costs... How customers cost their idle time may not always be calculable, but can sometimes be inferred by observation, for example, of the way in which customers will leave a queue to go elsewhere if they consider it to be too long or too slow.

In hospital queueing problems, costs are more difficult to define. What is the cost of keeping a patient waiting in the out-patient clinic? What is the cost of rejecting a patient requiring intensive care? In very few cases is it possible or even desirable to put these into money terms. However, methods are available for obtaining partial measures of these costs, and they are helpful when an operational solution is being sought. Even if we cannot quantify the costs and benefits they should be clearly described."

MATHEMATICAL SOLUTIONS

In general the length of queues will fluctuate but, hopefully, they will always be eventually reduced. A queuing system can be classified into one of three 'states':

(a)   a transient state where the system is working out the upsets of the initial queue formation.

(b)   if the average arrival rate is less than the average service rate (and both are constant) the system will eventually settle down to a steady state. The existence of the steady state does not imply that there will be no queues, nor that the length of the queue will be unvarying. It does imply, however, that the average waiting time, for example, will be constant even though successive customers may have to wait for different times.

(c)   If the average arrival rate is greater than the average service rate, the queue will get out of control and there will always be a queue which will simply get longer and longer. This situation is known as the explosive case.

If the queue is in a steady state, certain mathematical formulae are available to calculate the average number of people in the queue, the probability of the system being idle etc. A great deal of research has been undertaken in queuing theory but we shall be concentrating on one case: what is known as the M/M/1 queuing system. This is the case of the one channel queue with Poisson arrivals and negative exponential service times.

Queuing nomenclature

A standardised method of describing queuing models has been developed. (It is often called Kendall's notation.) Each model is described by three symbols: the first representing the arrival pattern; the second, the service pattern and the third, the number of servers.

The symbols used are as follows:

M   = negative exponential interarrival or service time (or Poisson arrivals). M is the abbreviation for Markovian.

D   = Deterministic, constant or regular.

E_n = Erlang distribution of order n.

G   = General distribution (i.e. a nonspecified distribution).

As indicated above, in the following discussion we will concentrate on M/M/1 i.e. Poisson arrivals, negative exponential service time and 1 server or channel. Other models may be M/M/S

(S servers); $E_n/M/1$ (Erlang arrivals, negative exponential service time, 1 channel) etc.

The M/M/1 System

Let us now consider a mathematical solution of a Poisson arrival, negative exponential service time system. We shall also assume that it is a one channel – single phase system. The Poisson distribution, you will recall is:

$$P(r) = \frac{e^{-\lambda}\lambda^r}{r!}$$

and the negative exponential is

$$y \quad = \mu e^{-\mu t}$$

with λ = arrival rate
μ = service rate

Given these distributions, and a steady state system a number of formulae have been derived. (The proofs of these formulae are complex but may be found in Wagner, 1969.)

(a) Traffic Intensity

A useful statistic is the traffic intensity: a measure of the extent to which the system is working to capacity.

The traffic intensity is normally denoted by ρ (rho) and is defined:

For an M/M/1 system, if $\rho > 1$, the system is in an explosive state. Obviously in the M/M/1 case the greater , the longer will be the average waiting time.

(b) Number in the system

There are a number of formulae relating to the number of people in a queuing system. First we could consider the probability that there are n people in the system. This is normally denoted by P_n (to distinguish it from P(r) – the probability that there are r arrivals in any unit of time).

Now

$$P_n = (1 - \frac{\lambda}{\mu}) \; (\frac{\lambda}{\mu})^n$$

Note that this formula yields the probability of a given number in the system: i.e. the number waiting (or the number in the queue) plus the number being served. This difference in the formulae between the system and the queue is an important one.

Example 3.2

If the average arrival rate of patients to the booking clerks in an outpatients department is .3 per minute and the average service rate .7 per minute, what are the probabilities of the various numbers of people in the system?

Now $\lambda = .3$

$\mu = .7$

hence $P_n = (1 - \frac{\lambda}{\mu}) \, (\frac{\lambda}{\mu})^n$

$= (1 - \frac{.3}{.7}) \, (\frac{.3}{.7})^n$

$= (1 - .428) \, (.428)^n$

$= .571 \times (.428)^n$ (to nearest three decimal places)

Now if $n = 0$

$P_0 = .571 \times (.428)^0$

$= .571$ (since $.428^0 = 1$ by definition)

for $n = 1$

$P_1 = (.571) \times .428$

$= .244$

and for other n,

$P_2 = .104$

$P_3 = .044$

$P_4 = .019$

$P_5 = .008$

$P_6 = .003$

Now the sum of all the P_n is 1 since the P_n are probabilities;

and $P_0 + P_1 + P_2 + P_3 + P_4 + P_5 + P_6 = \sum\limits_{n=0}^{6} P_n = .993$

then $\sum\limits_{n=7}^{\infty} P_n = 1 - .993$

$= .007$

and hence the probability that there is more than six people in the system is .007.

Idle Time

One important statistic derived from the number of patients in the system is that concerning the probability of there being no people in the system. Clearly if there are no people in the system the facility is idle. The proportion of idle time is then found by setting $n = 0$ in the formula for the number in the system.

Hence

Probability of there being 0 people in the system

= probability of the system being idle

$= P_o = (1 - \frac{\lambda}{\mu}) \ (\frac{\lambda}{\mu})^n$

$= (1 - \frac{\lambda}{\mu}) \ (\frac{\lambda}{\mu})^0$

$= (1 - \frac{\lambda}{\mu})$ by definition.

In example 3.2 above the proportion of idle time would be 57.1%. Note that idle time <u>decreases</u> as traffic intensity increases.

The second statistic relating to the number in the system is the <u>expected (average or mean) number in the system</u>. This is comonly denoted L and is derived by use of the following formula:

$$L = \frac{\lambda}{\mu - \lambda}$$

Example 3.3

If $\lambda = .3$ and $\mu = .7$ what is the expected number in the system?

$$L = \frac{.3}{.7 - .3}$$

$$= \frac{.3}{.4}$$

$$= .75$$

(c) <u>Other statistics</u>

Two important statistics can be calculated concerning the queue.

(i)   Expected waiting time in the <u>queue</u>

$$= \frac{\cdot \lambda}{\mu(\mu - \lambda)}$$

(ii)   Expected (average) number in the <u>queue</u>

$$= \frac{\lambda^2}{\mu(\mu - \lambda)}$$

It is important to note that both these statistics can be found once the service rate and the arrival rate are known. As a corollary of this it should be noted that if the waiting time is to be altered either the service rate or the arrival rate must be altered (and, of course, arrival rate may be uncontrollable!).

Example 3.4

Assuming Poisson arrivals averaging .3 per minute and exponential service time averaging 85 seconds (.7 per minute) what is

(i)   the expected number of customers who would be waiting at any given time

and (ii)   the average length of time they would wait in the queue.

(i) Average waiting time

$$= \frac{\lambda}{\mu(\mu-\lambda)}$$
$$= \frac{.3}{.7(.7-.3)}$$
$$= \frac{.3}{.28}$$
$$= 1.07$$

i.e. The average waiting time would be 1 minute 4.2 seconds.

(ii) Expected number in the queue

$$= \frac{\lambda^2}{\mu(\mu-\lambda)}$$
$$= \frac{(.3)^2}{.7(.7-.3)}$$
$$= \frac{.09}{.7 \times .4}$$
$$= \frac{.09}{.28}$$
$$= .321$$

Formulae & Tables

We have concentrated on the simplest queuing system: an M/M/1 system with one phase. Few real-life systems are that simple. We have also concentrated on the simplest formulae of the M/M/1 system: mean number in the queue, mean waiting time etc. However, formulae have been derived for the more complex indicators of queue performance and for the more complex queuing systems. For instance, formulae exist for the probability that a customer would have to wait less than t units of time and for the mean waiting time in an M/M/S queuing system (see Eiselt & von Frajer, 1977).

Solving Queuing Problems

As with all operations research problems there is clearly a balance to be struck - this time it is between the cost of providing the service and the cost of not providing the service or only providing a given level of service (and if not providing or only providing at a given level, costs of increased waiting time). Thus, for example, the administrator of a hospital may be concerned with minimising the proportion of time during which the facility is idle bearing in mind that the less idle time there is the greater the probability of long queues.

As with inventory models, the measurement of costs again would present a problem especially when one attempts to measure the cost of customer waiting time. However, as in all resources allocation problems, there are costs associated with providing a given level of service and there are costs associated with not providing that service. The administrator must work towards an optimal situation where costs are minimised subject to a policy on the level of service to be offered.

Thus, for example, a hospital board may decide that no one will ever wait for treatment in the emergency facilities and a given

number of medical practitioners will have to be allocated to
provide this service. On the other hand, the board may accept an
average waiting time of 40 minutes so the doctors can be utilized
elsewhere. It is often the case, however, that administrators
either say that a perfect level of service must be provided
(regardless of cost) or ignore completely the fact that different
levels of service can be provided. Similarly hospital
administrators will often shrug their shoulders and say that a
situation is subject to such random variations that nothing can
be done, yet it has been shown (Newell 1954, 1964) that whenever
the average number of emergency admissions is between 1 and 30,
if 2 beds more than the average are held for ·emergencies, demand
will be satisfied in 95% of all cases. But, of course, this is
not the final answer: what effect does the 'mean plus two'
policy have on utilization? As was indicated above a queuing
system involves an inherent trade off: between idle time (or
utilization) of providers and waiting time of patients.

The result of a study of Rising (1977) illustrates this point.

Figure 3.7 illustrates how provider utilization and patient
waiting change with the change in the number of providers.
Rising describes it thus:

"In this simplified example, the outpatient facility normally
operates 8 hours per day with three physicians who see about
170 patients per day; all the patients are walk-ins, and all
providers are available throughout clinic works.

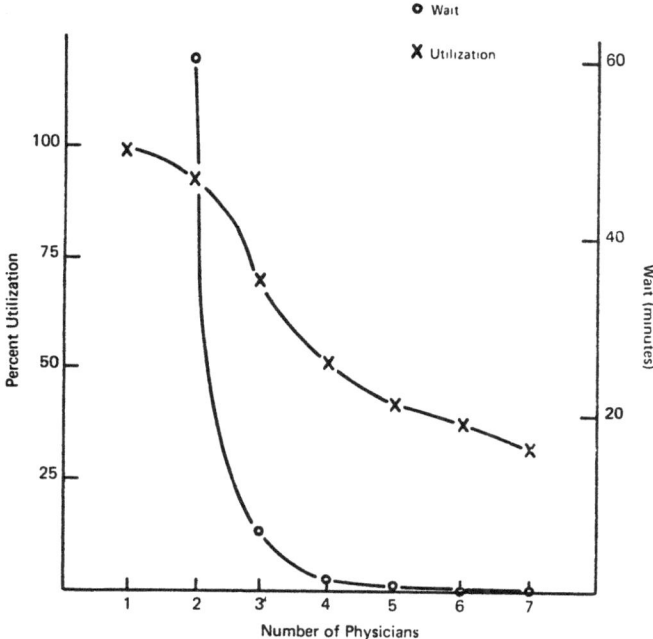

<u>Figure 3.7</u>   The Effect of Changing the Number of Physicians in a
Hypothetical Clinic on the Patient Waiting Time and
Physician Utilization.

Figure 3.7 shows that the use of three physicians in this situation results in a utilization of about 70 percent and an average patient wait of about 14 minutes; also it clearly shows that any attempt to increase the physician utilization will cause an increase in patient waiting time, and vice versa. Further examination of Figure 3.7 shows that the utilization would be increased from the current 70 percent to about 95 percent if one of the physicians were removed or happened to be absent for any reason; however, this also causes an increase in the average patient waiting time from under 14 minutes to over 60 minutes. On the other hand, the patient waiting time can be reduced from 14 minutes to under 4 minutes by adding an extra physician, but the consequence of this change is a reduction of physician utilization from the current value of 70 percent to under 52 percent.

Scheduling of Arrivals

It has been shown above that the existence of queues, and hence the presence of the waiting costs, is in part a consequence of the random distribution of arrivals. Thus as an alternative to increasing the size or number of service facilities it may be possible to reduce the size of queues by scheduling the arrival of customers. For given arrival and service rates, exercise of control over the system in such a way that arrivals are evenly spaced over time will invariably reduce the average size of queues which form.

Whether it is possible to schedule arrivals depends, of course, on the circumstances associated with the specific queuing situation. It is obviously not possible to induce bank or cafeteria customers to seek service at predetermined times, or to ensure that equipment only breaks down on the hour. However, it is quite feasible to schedule the arrival of aircraft at an airport, and to introduce an appointments system in a hospital outpatients department! It is also possible for hospitals to attempt to influence the arrival rate during "crisis" periods by, say, encouraging potential patients to ring to check what is the current waiting time. Scheduling systems are discussed in more detail in Rising (1977, Chapter 4).

APPLICATIONS

Of the many areas in which queues develop, two shall be considered.

(1) Inpatient Facilities

Thompson used queuing models to analyse the operation of a maternity unit at the Yale New Haven Hospital (Thompson et al, 1959, 1963). Upon admission patients were cared for in the labor room, delivery room etc. Thompson plotted the distribution of service times in each stage of care and discovered that service times (i.e. length of stay) were distributed negative exponentially. The arrival rate was, subject to minor seasonal and temporal variations, distributed according to the Poisson distribution. A multi channel model was used to determine predicted frequencies of use of between 0 & 5 delivery rooms, these were then checked with actual experience.

Table 3.2 Usage of Delivery Rooms

No. of Patients Using Delivery Rooms	Queuing Prediction	Actual Experience
0	.6413	.6118
1	.2849	.2983
2	.0633	.0802
3	.0094	.0069
4	.0010	.0024
5	.0001	.0004

The difference between the actual and the predicted was important and apparently lies in the deviation of arrivals from the true Poisson distribution (some scheduling takes place and arrivals are not truly random).

(2) Outpatient Facilities

Treatment in an outpatient clinic or in a casualty department/emergency room yields classic queuing theory problems. In most ambulatory emergency situations patients walk in off the street and request that they be seen by a medical practitioner. They may or may not have to wait. Having been seen, they may also require radiology in which case a further wait may be necessary. Eventually, however, they will be treated and depart.

An example of the application of queuing theory in an outpatient setting may be found in Rising et al (1973). In this example a queuing model of an outpatient department which treats between 400 and 500 patients per day was derived. The inter-arrival time of patients was plotted and is shown in Figure 3.8.

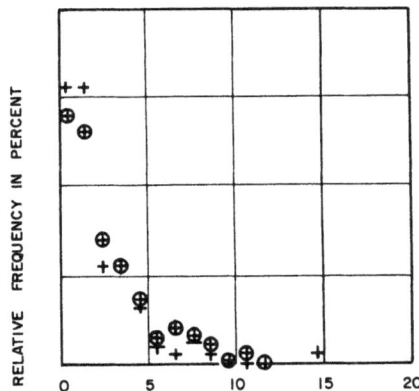

PATIENT INTER-ARRIVAL TIME IN MINUTES

Fig. 3.8. The frequency distribution of patient interarrival times. + Monday, April 6, 1970; x=2.167, s=2.402, n=237. ⊕ Thursday, April 9, 1970; x=2.626, s=2.8338, n=202.

Values are plotted for a Monday and a Thursday and both allow for
the assumption of a negative exponential distribution.   Monday
and Thursday were used because the University of Massachusetts
schedules lectures in blocks on Monday, Wednesday and Friday and
on Tuesday and Thursday and so the two days are plotted to
identify any biasing effect of the timetabling arrangement.   The
patients arriving at the clinic fell into three groups: those
with appointments; walk-in patients and patients being called
back for a second visit.   The distribution of the relative
frequency of service times for second-visit patients is shown in
Figure 3.9.

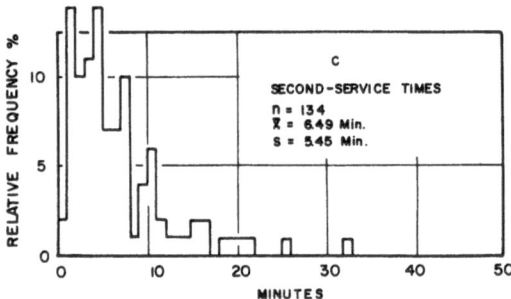

PATIENT SERVICE TIMES IN MINUTES

Figure 3.9

The study is a well written description of a study of a queuing
process, and it can be seen from the two Figures the relevance of
the assumption of negative exponential inter-arrival times
(Poisson arrivals) and service times.

Nine Elements of Queuing Problems

It was suggested earlier in this unit that all queuing systems
contain nine common elements.   Table 3.3 summarises these for the
inpatient and outpatient applications.

Table 3.3 Comparison of Queuing Applications

Element	Inpatient Facility	Outpatient Facility
Facility	Obstetric Suite	Emergency Room
Customer	Pregnant Patient	Patient
Server	Delivery Room Bed	Attending Physician
Arrival Pattern	Poisson	Possibly Poisson for similar time periods (i.e. 10 pm – 6 am) with different arrival rates for different periods
Service Pattern	Negative Exponential	Negative Exponential
Queue Discipline	First Come First Served	Some Urgent Others First Come First Served
Arrangement of Services	In parallel (Possibly in series for use of post partum care)	Single server or in parallel
Customer Cost	+ve (cost) *Delivery in inadequate conditions *inconvenience *anxiety	+ve *deterioration of condition *inconvenience *monetary loss (work absenteeism)
	−ve (benefit) *Delivery of baby	−ve *probable improvement in condition
Service Cost	+ve Capital Costs, Salaries	+ve Capital Costs, Salaries
	+ve or −ve Community Goodwill	+ve or − ve Goodwill

It can quickly be seen that both examples are typical queuing problems. It should be noted that it is possible to put valuations on all of the above elements and the problem of the level of service to be supplied can then be solved mathematically.

LIMITATIONS OF MATHEMATICAL QUEUING MODELS

Although queuing systems are quite common in hospitals, queuing theory is only used infrequently as a solution to the problems at hand. The major factor which reduces the use of mathematical

queuing models is the requirement that mathematical
representations of arrival and service patterns be obtained.
Although the Poisson distribution has been used in a number of
studies, any scheduling of arrivals (such as the introduction of
an appointments system) will immediately invalidate the use of
the Poisson. Yet despite the introduction of appointment
systems, patients still wait in the Outpatients Department!

Another factor which reduces the applicability of mathematical
models is a neglect of behavioural implications. The behaviour
of physicians seeing patients, for example, may vary with the
length of the queue! (Rockart and Hoffman (1969) showed that if
only a few patients were waiting physicians would spend more time
with each patient.)

Queuing models do not, of course, normally take into accout the
host of factors which affect their application. The hospital may
not be able to schedule arrivals; it may not be possible to
produce reliable estimates of service time and it is generally
not possible to influence the behaviour of the physician (who
determines much of the success of any system introduced).

SUMMARY AND CONCLUSION

Wherever a service is provided and is demanded, customers will
arrive at the service point and may have to wait. These rates of
arrival may be able to be predicted (within certain limits) and
the amount of time it takes for them to pass through the system
may also be predictable. The resulting queues and idle time are
of interest to management. Queuing theory has been developed to
attempt to determine how service points should be organised, how
many people should be there to serve etc.

Queuing models have certain readily recognisable characteristics
and can be applied to many different areas of hospital
administration. The application is limited, however, by the need
to develop mathematical relationships for certain variables.
Mitchell (1972) however, notes:

"These various limitations of queuing theory have meant that
simulation has become very widely used as a means of studying
queuing situations. It would, however, be wrong to dismiss
queuing theory. In the first place there are plenty of
situations of importance where the assumptions queuing theory
makes and therefore the results of applying it are valid.
Certainly if it can be used it is to be preferred to
simulation as the cheaper and more accurate method.

In addition, and perhaps more importantly, queuing theory
provides models which are good enough in a great many cases
to give useful insight into the system under study and into
how it might be improved."

REFERENCES

Eiselt, H.A. & von Frajer, H. (1977) Operations Research Handbook: Standard Algorithms & Methods with Examples, Walter de Gruter.

Hollingdale, S.H. (1978) 'Methods of Operational Analysis' in Lighthill, J. (ed) Newer Uses of Mathematics, Penguin.

Jones, G.T. (1972) Simulation & Business Decisions, Penguin.

Luck, G.M., Luckman, J., Smith, B.W. & Stringer, J. (1971) Patients, Hospitals, and Operational Research, Tavistock.

Mitchell, G.H. (ed) (1972) Operational Research: Techniques & Examples, English Uni. Press.

Newell, D.J. (1964). 'Immediate admissions to hospital', Proceedings of the 3rd International Conference on Operational Research, pp. 224-233, London.

Newell, D.J. (1954) 'Provision of emergency beds in hospitals', British Journal of Preventive and Social Medicine, 8 (App), pp. 77-80.

Rising, E.J. (1977) Ambulatory Care Systems Vol 1: Design for Improved Patient Flow, Lexington.

Rising, E.J., Baron, R. & Averill, B. (1973) 'A Systems Analysis of a University Health Service Outpatient Clinic', Operations Research, Vol. 21, No. 5, pp. 1030-1047.

Rockart, J.R. & Hoffman, P.B. (1969) 'Physician & patient behaviour under different scheduling systems in hospital outpatient departments', Medical Care, Vol 7, pp. 463-470.

Thompson, J.D. et al (1963) 'Predicting Requirements for maternity Facilities', Hospitals, February 16.

Thompson, J.D. et al (1959) 'Yale Studies of Hospital Function and Design', unpublished 1959 study described in Griffith, J.R. Quantitative Techniques for Hospital Planning & Control, Heath Lexington.

Wagner, H.M. (1969) Principles of Operations Research, Prentice Hall.

Warner, D.M. & Holloway, D.C. (1978) Decision Making & Control for Health Administration: The Management of Quantitative Analysis, Health Administration Press.

QUEUING SUMMARY

ELEMENTS OF QUEUING PROBLEMS

1. There is a FACILITY providing service

2. There are CUSTOMERS who arrive to use the facility

3. There are SERVERS who provide service

4. The customers arrive in a certain a PATTERN

    We assume the ARRIVAL PATTERN is distributed according to the POISSON distribution: Arrivals are random in the sense that the probability of an arrival in any unit of time is independent of the number of arrivals in any previous unit of time; Poisson also implies that the time beteen arrivals is distributed according to a negative exponential distribution.

    Relevant Formula:

    P(r arrivals in any unit of time) =

    $$\frac{e^{-\lambda}\lambda^{r}}{r!}$$

5. The customers are served in a particular pattern. We assume that frequency of service times are distributed negative exponentially, i.e. most customers require only a short service time whilst a few require a very long service time.

    Relevant Formula:

    Frequency of Service Time $= \mu e^{-\mu t}$
    μ = Service rate

6. There is a QUEUE DISCIPLINE

7. The servers are ARRANGED

8. There is a CUSTOMER COST

9. There is a SERVICE COST

MATHEMATICAL SOLUTION OF QUEUING PROBLEMS

Number in System: $P_n = (1 - \frac{\lambda}{\mu})(\frac{\lambda}{\mu})^n$

Special Case (n≠0) $P_0 = (1 - \frac{\lambda}{\mu})$

Expected number in Queue $= \dfrac{\lambda^2}{\mu(\mu-\lambda)}$

Expected waiting time in Queue $= \dfrac{\lambda}{\mu(\mu-\lambda)}$

4   SIMULATION

In many cases exact mathematical representations of queuing systems are inappropriate for there may be no mathematical distribution that can be assumed to represent arrivals or service times. Bus timetables or scheduling of patients may preclude the use of queuing formulae. Similarly, the interaction of a number of variables in an inventory may be extremely complex and it may be difficult to formulate an optimum inventory policy.

A technique known as simulation is available which can assist decision makers to make choices in situations such as these. Like most operations research techniques, simulation involves building a model which is a representation of reality and manipulating the variables to assess the effect of different policies or different scenarios. Simulation, however, does not rely on mathematical formulae to provide estimates of system variables such as waiting time but rather, such variables are produced as a result of a series of iterations undertaken as part of the simulation process.

The essence of simulation is that it mirrors or repeats real life situations and allows direct calculation of system statistics. Thus a simulation model might have portrayed the number of arrivals to a queuing system in a 100 minutes on 100 consecutive lines of paper. Using the number of lines as an analogy to the number of minutes, one can calculate certain queue statistics by inspection (e.g. the probability of zero arrivals in any unit of time is found by adding up the number of lines with no arrival recorded and dividing that by 100).

It is often easier to build a model which simulates arrival rates and service time in a way that represents real life rather than attempt to force arrivals or service time distributions into mathematical distributions that are inappropriate. By a series of experiments with a simple model we can thus derive the various queue statistics such as percentage idle time and average waiting time. Similarly modifications to the model can be made to take account of, say, unacceptable queue lengths.

Hollingdale (1978, pp.249-250) described simulation as follows:

> "The technique is to create, and trace through over a period of time, a typical 'life history' of the system under prescribed conditions... The effect of variability on the system as a whole is reproduced by 'sampling' from the appropriate probability distributions. These may be derived from frequency distributions, observations (or 'counts') of how the system has behaved in the past, or may be

distributions specified directly by mathematical functions, or a mixture of both. This rather 'brute force' aproach necessarily entails a lot of calculation and data processing and (is) a situation where the use of computers is essential to the effective exploitation of a technique."

One of the great merits of simulation is that it enables the effects of changes in the system to be assessed by experimenting with the model instead of with the system itself. This not only yields obvious advantages in terms of cost and convenience, but in many cases it is the only practicable way to proceed. A manager cannot choose a sales plan for next year by trying out all the possibilities this year. An airport controller cannot determine the effect of a 25% increase of traffic by direct experiment. There are many situations in which a decision-maker must either rely on his 'hunch' or seek assistance from digital simulation experiments conducted on a simplified model of the actual system."

The essence of simulation then is that manipulation of a mathematical model allows the decision maker to draw conclusions about a system, and about the effect of changes to the system.

Gaver (1978) described the general steps involved in a simulation study:

"(1)   Problem definition: identification of the important issues.

(2)   Empirical information collection and data analysis; establishment of client contact.

(3)   Model formulation: agreement upon abstractions, acceptable simplifiations, and relevant responses and measures of performance.

(4)   Model construction or selection: documentation of sub-models, and parameter determination.

(5)   Model manipulation: computations to determine responses when model conditions vary; experimental design and 'variance reduction'.

(6)   Validation studies: is computational outcome in conformity with input (e.g. are programming errors present) and is computational outcome consistent with 'real world' experience?

(7)   Communication of results to client: replay of parts of the above, depending upon what is learned."

The first stages of the simulation process are extremely important. We have to define clearly the problem and ensure that we collect all relevant information. Any simulation model we eventually develop will only produce relevant results if an adequate range of accurate data has been used as input. However, we shall concentrate here on steps 4 and 5: Model construction and manipulation.

Model Construction and Manipulation

All uses of operations research involve model building and simulation is no exception.

Having defined our problem, and collected data the next step in the simulation model is to construct a model to represent the reality we are investigating. In some circumstances this may involve a mathematical distribution (e.g. we could develop a simulation model of a outpatient clinic system which involves a mathematical distribution of arrivals) or alternatively we may choose to represent arrivals by a probability distribution based on the observed arrival pattern which does not follow any known distribution. Both the probabilities and the mathematical distribution would be derived from an analysis of the data we had collected during the previous stages.

This model construction stage can be quite complex - especially if we are modelling a complex process. Thus a simulation model of a hospital might involve a number of components (e.g. a simulation of operating theatres) and would probably be facilitated if we had designed a diagram (sometimes called a flow chart) to specify the interdependencies in the model.

The next step in the simulation process is to manipulate the model. In most simulations this involves use of random numbers. Basically, the various outcomes specified in our probability distribution are allocated a set of numbers in proportion to the probability of the occurrence of that outcome. (This process is called association of outcomes.) Thus if we had undertaken a survey and found that in 20% of the cases (of clients attending a clinic) the service time was 20 minutes, then we would allocate 20% of the numbers from which we are sampling to represent clients with a service time of 20 minutes. We normally record this association process sequentially as it is easier to keep a record of which numbers have been allocated to represent which event.

A sampling procedure is then undertaken to simulate events (i.e. arrivals or time periods etc.) using random numbers from tables or using a random number generator. This process is repeated for a number of events and the statistics are than calculated from the model.

The model construction and manipulation phases thus involve the following steps:

1. Derivation of the probability distribution of the various outcomes.

2. Association of the various outcomes with certain numbers. Having determined the probability of an occurrence, that proportion of the numbers we are sampling from would be set aside to indicate that outcome.

3. Using a table of random numbers (or a 'random number' generator), a sampling procedure is used to stimulate a certain time period or series of events.

4. Statistics are generated by averaging the results of the
    simulation.

These steps are normally followed in every simulation, more
complex simulations may involve steps 1, 2 & 3 being repeated.
The examples below show the use of these steps in simple and more
complex simulations.

Example 4.1   THE NEWSPAPER SELLER PROBLEM

Let us assume that a newspaper seller buys papers from a
newsagent at 5¢ each and sells them at 8¢ each. Although there
is no monetary cost associated with failure to provide enough
papers to meet the day's demand (other than the profit foregone),
the seller receives no payment for any papers left over at the
end of the day. The problem is to determine how many papers the
seller should obtain from the newsagent each day.

As a good manager our newspaper seller has maintained records of
sales over the last 100 days. The results are as follows:

Table 4.1   Frequency Distribution of Newspapers Sold

No. of Papers Sold	No. of Days
20	1
21	3
22	8
23	12
24	16
25	19
26	13
27	9
28	10
29	5
30	4
	100

Thus it can be seen that on one day 20 papers were sold, on three
of the preceding 100 days, 21 papers were sold etc.

Having stated the problem and collected the data we now enter the
model construction and model manipulation phases. The problem is
simple: the newspaper seller is faced with determining the
optimum stock level. Importantly, demand does not follow any
particular mathematical distribution. A number of options are
open to the seller, including:

1. Always supplying the modal demand (25).
2. Ensuring that the mean demand (26) is always satisfied.
3. Following a variable decision rule, such as supplying
    one more paper than was demanded the previous day.

Simulation can be used to test out the profitability of each of
these decision rules. We shall follow the steps outlined
previously.

Step 1:   Derivation of the probability distribution of the
            outcomes

From the data in Table 4.1 we can derive a probability
distribution of the number of customers who will demand
newspapers. This is shown in Table 4.2 and is simply column 2 of
Table 4.1 expressed as a probability distribution.

Table 4.2 Probability Distribution of Number of Customers

Customers	Probability
20	.01
21	.03
22	.08
23	.12
24	.16
25	.19
26	.13
27	.09
28	.10
29	.05
30	.04
	1.00

Step 2: Association of the outcomes

The next step is to allocate a certain proportion of the sampling
frame (or numbers from which we will be sampling) to represent
these outcomes.   Thus, if we are going to be using a table of
random numbers which lie between 00 and 99 (i.e. 100 numbers in
all), we will allocate the relevant proportion of those 100
numbers to each outcome. Table 4.3 shows this process.

Table 4.3 Allocation of Numbers to Outcomes

Number of customers	Probability	Number of numbers to be allocated	Actual sequential numbers allocated
20	.01	1	00
21	.03	3	01-03
22	.08	8	04-11
23	.12	12	12-23
24	.16	16	24-39
25	.19	19	40-58
26	.13	13	59-71
27	.09	9	72-80
28	.10	10	81-90
29	.05	5	91-95
30	.04	4	96-99
	1.00	100	

It can be seen that 20 papers will be sold on one day (i.e.
probability of occurrence is .01 we are sampling from 100 numbers
and so .01 x 100 = 1 number will be allocated) and we represent
20 sales by one number. It is easiest to allocate the numbers to
represent the particular outcomes on a sequential basis so we
allocate the number 00 to represent 20 sales. Now 21 sales are
made on three days (probability of occurrence .03, .03 x 100 =
3) and so we represent 21 sales by three numbers, specifically
the next three available numbers, 01, 02, and 03. This procedure
is repeated for each level of sales and as there are only records
for 100 days, each number between 00 and 99 will have one and
only one level of sales assigned to it.

Step 3: Use of random numbers

Having allocated the numbers from the sampling frame, we can now
use a table of random numbers to represent the experience of the
chance event: the demand for newspapers. Random number tables
are included in a number of text books and an example of the
random number table for numbers between 00 and 99 is included as
Table 4.4.

Table 4.4   Random Numbers Between 00 & 99

55	59	30
84	90	70
67	52	40
05	38	03
00	03	15
29	54	81
25	87	06
83	02	87
72	21	98
95	92	24

The numbers allocated in Table 4.3 lie between 00 and 99 and so
Table 4.4 can be used as a sampling frame. The random numbers
are used to represent the various outcomes. The first random
number, 55, is thus used to represent the sale of 25 newspapers
(from Table 4.3 since 55 lies between 40 and 58 it has been
allocated to 25 sales). The second random number, 84 represents
28 sales (from Table 4.3 since 84 lies between 81 and 90). We
can thus simulate a number of days experience for each of the
possible policy options. In most actual uses of simulation a
large number of 'days' or trials are made and the actual events
recorded will occur in accordance (and closely approximating)
their specified probabilities.

Using the random numbers of Table 4.4 as our sample, and the
association rules given in Table 4.3, we can now simulate the
profit patterns for various decision rules.

Table 4.5 shows the results for following decision rule 1 (i.e.
always supplying the modal demand (25)). Column 1 shows the
random number; Column 2, the demand that number represents;
Column 3, the newspapers supplied (following decision rule 1,
this a constant); Column 4, the number of newspapers returned;

Column 5, is the net profit that day and Column 6, the cumulative profit.

Table 4.5 Simulation of Newspaper Seller Problem

Random Number	Simulated Demand	Newspapers provided	Returns	Net Profit	Cumulative Profit
55	25	25	–	75	.75
84	28	25	–	75	1.50
67	26	25	–	75	2.25
05	22	25	3	51	2.76
00	20	25	5	35	3.11
29	24	25	1	67	3.78
25	24	25	1	67	4.45
83	28	25	–	75	5.20
72	27	25	–	75	5.95
95	29	25	–	75	6.70

One would normally simulate each decision rule for a large number of trials (days) before a clear pattern could emerge. Having done this for each of the decision rules, it would then be possible to select the strategy which yields the maximum profit.

The newspaper sales problem is the simplest of all simulation models, it involves simulation of one variable only (sales); and is only slightly more complicated if one simulates different decision rules.

Simulation methods can handle much more complicated systems, as the next example shows.

Example 4.2 EMERGENCY CLINICS

Assume that the Putney Hospital conducts an emergency clinic which sees a couple of people every hour. Although the administrator is happy with the average waiting time of patients, she is not satisfied with the level of 'idle time'. She plans to simulate the system, however, before changing the rostering system for medical officers. Again the first stages of the process involve problem definition and data collection. We can assume that this has been done. We now commence the model construction and model manipulation phases. Our model is a simple queuing one:

Arrivals   Queue   Service   Departure

Figure 4.1 Model of Casualty Problem

Our next stages replicate the newspaper sales problem and the standard steps of the model manipulation phase. This time, however, steps 1, 2 & 3 are repeated.

1) Derivation of probability distribution

Let us assume that the arrivals and service times can be
represented according to the probability distributions shown in
Tables 4.6 and 4.7.

Table 4.6 Distribution of Arrivals

Number of arrivals per hour	Probability
0	.1
1	.1
2	.3
3	.4
4	.1
	1.0

(Note that the expected arrival rate is 2.3 per hour.)

Table 4.7 Distribution of Service Times

Service time in minutes	Probability
5	.05
10	.20
15	.50
20	.25
	1.00

Note that the expected service time is 14.75 minutes and thus
60/14.75 services are provided per hour i.e. the service rate
is approximately 4 per hour. As the service rate is greater than
the arrival rate, a steady state situation will emerge and we can
proceed with the simulation.

As mentioned above, we have to repeat steps 2 & 3. We will first
work through steps 2 & 3 simulating the arrivals.

2) Association of the outcomes-for arrivals

We can again use a sampling frame of the 100 numbers between 00
and 99 for arrivals. Table 4.8 shows the association process.

Table 4.8 Allocation of Numbers to Arrivals

Arrivals per hour	Probability	Numbers of numbers to be allocated	Sequential numbers allocated
0	.1	10	00-09
1	.1	10	10-19
2	.3	30	20-49
3	.4	40	50-89
4	.1	10	90-99
	1.0	100	

It can be seen that generation of Table 4.8 follows the same procedures as were used earlier. Column 2 shows the probability of a given number of arrivals taken from Table 4.6; Column 3 shows the number of random numbers that we would allocate (as we are sampling from 100 numbers, .1 x 100 = 10 numbers would be used to represent 0 arrivals and so on); Column 4 shows the actual numbers allocated.

3) Use of Random Numbers - for arrivals

Having allocated our numbers we can use a table of random numbers to replicate or simulate the arrivals. Table 4.9 shows the first part of this process.

Table 4.9   Simulated Arrivals for First 30 Hours

Period	Random Number	Arrivals
1	55	3
2	84	3
3	67	3
4	05	0
5	00	0
6	29	2
7	25	2
8	83	3
9	72	3
10	95	4
11	59	3
12	90	4
13	52	3
14	38	2
15	03	0
16	54	3
17	87	3
18	02	0
19	21	2
20	92	4
21	30	2
22	70	3
23	46	2
24	03	0
25	15	1
26	81	3
27	06	0
82	87	3
92	98	4
30	24	2

Note that the first column is the period (or hour) being simulated. The second column shows the random number taken from Table 4.4. Column 3 shows the number of arrivals in that hour as represented by the relevant random number thus, in the first hour, the number of arrivals is represented by the random number 55 which falls between 50 and 88 in Table 4.8 and hence implies 3 arrivals.

In the absence of any other information and for simplicity one could assume that the arrivals are spread evenly over the hour – so the three arrivals in time period 1 would occur at 20, 40 and 60 minutes after the hour (i.e. the last arrival occurs at the beginning of the next hour). The two arrivals in time period 6 would occur under this assumption at 30 and 60 minutes. Another spacing arrangement of arrivals would be to assume that they are evenly spaced within the hour. That is for one arrival, this takes place after 30 minutes of the hour have elapsed. For 2 arrivals, these take place after 20 and 40 minutes respectively. We shall assume that it is this latter pattern that prevails. A further option would be to have recourse to another set of random numbers to determine the spacing of arrivals.

Table 4.10 Simulated Arrivals for Time Period 31 to 200

Period	Arrivals	Period	Arrivals	Period	Arrivals	Period	Arrivals	Period	Arrivals	Period	Arrivals
31	3	61	4	91	2	121	4	151	1	180	2
32	1	62	2	92	1	122	1	152	2	181	3
33	2	63	1	93	2	123	4	153	3	182	1
34	2	64	3	94	2	124	2	154	1	183	3
35	2	65	2	95	3	125	3	155	3	184	2
36	2	66	2	96	4	126	3	156	3	185	3
37	0	67	3	97	1	127	3	157	3	186	3
38	3	68	0	98	1	128	2	158	3	187	2
39	3	69	2	99	3	129	3	159	2	188	2
40	3	70	0	100	3	130	3	160	2	189	2
41	2	71	4	101	3	131	3	161	1	190	2
42	2	72	3	102	3	132	2	162	2	191	1
43	2	73	3	103	3	133	1	163	2	192	3
44	3	74	3	104	2	134	0	164	3	193	3
45	2	75	2	105	4	135	3	165	2	194	2
46	3	76	2	106	2	136	3	166	1	195	2
47	3	77	2	107	2	137	2	167	3	196	3
48	2	78	3	108	3	138	3	168	2	197	2
49	0	79	0	109	3	139	2	169	3	198	0
50	3	80	2	110	0	140	3	170	0	199	4
51	2	81	3	111	3	141	1	171	3	200	0
52	3	82	3	112	4	142	1	172	2		
53	3	83	3	113	4	143	3	173	2		
54	3	84	2	114	2	144	3	174	2		
55	2	85	3	115	3	145	1	175	2		
56	0	86	2	116	2	146	2	176	2		
57	3	87	2	117	0	147	3	177	1		
58	2	88	0	118	1	148	1	178	3		
59	2	89	4	119	3	149	3	179	3		
60	2	90	3	120	4	150	1				

Table 4.10 shows the number of simulated arrivals for the next 170 hours, i.e. up to the 200th hour. Note that the random numbers are not included here although in practice it would be simple to show them for each time period.

For the 200 hours shown in Tables 4.9 and 4.10 the percentages of each number of arrivals are as follows:

Table 4.11 Frequency Distribution for Simulated 200 Arrivals

Number of arrivals per period	Frequency	Percentage
0	19	9.5 (10.0)
1	21	10.5 (10.0)
2	69	34.5 (30.0)
3	76	38.0 (40.0)
4	15	7.5 (10.0)
	200	100.0 100.0

The figures in brackets are the theoretical frequencies derived from the original probability distribution of arrivals shown in Table 4.6. It is seen that the agreement is reasonably close. If more than 200 periods had been simulated this sampling variability would be further reduced.

This example is somewhat more complex than the newspaper sales problem because two sampling exercises must be undertaken. Having sampled and estimated arrivals we must now estimate the service time distribution for each of those arrivals. Exactly the same steps are followed.

4) Repeating step 2, Association of the outcomes - for service times

Examination of Table 4.7, and application of principles of determining probabilities, determining the number of random numbers to be allocated and then allocating sequential numbers allows us to allocate the random numbers to represent the various service times shown in Table 4.12.

Table 4.12 Allocation of Numbers for Service Times

Service time in minutes	Probability	Numbers to be allocated	Sequential numbers allocated
5	.05	5	00-24
10	.20	20	05-24
15	.50	50	25-74
20	.25	25	75-99

Note that in this case each random number is used to indicate a
service time. This has implications for our sampling procedure
as we will draw a new number to represent the service time for
each arrival rather than for each time period.

5) Repeating step 3, Use of Random Numbers - for service times

If we are undertaking two sampling procedures for a single
simulation, we would normally use two separate series of random
numbers. We would follow the standard practice of drawing a
random number (say 78) and, using Table 4.12 we would record this
arrival as having a service time of 20 minutes. This process
would be repeating for each of the arrivals represented in Tables
4.9 and 4.10.

Thus as there were three arrivals in period i, three random
numbers would be drawn giving three service times. The results
for the first thirty time periods are shown in Table 4.13.

Table 4.13   Simulated Service Times

Period	Time (minutes)	Period	Times (minutes)
1	20, 15, 15	16	10, 15, 20
2	10, 15, 20	17	15, 15, 15
3	15, 15, 15	18	-
4	-	19	15, 15
5	-	20	20, 10, 15, 10
6	20, 5	21	20, 15
7	20, 20	22	20, 20, 20
8	15, 10, 10	23	10, 15
9	15, 20, 15	24	-
10	15, 20, 15, 10	25	15
11	20, 20, 20	26	15, 15, 20
12	15, 10, 15, 10	27	-
13	20, 15, 10	28	15, 20, 20
14	15, 10	29	15, 15, 15, 15
15	-	30	20, 10

Having simulated both arrival time and service distribution we
can now proceed to the final stages of the simulation.

6) Step 4 - Statistics of the System

Our administrator's objective would be to calculate simple queue
statistics for the system. These can be calculated by combining
the simulated arrivals and their associated service times and
assessing the effect on the system. Table 4.14 shows the first
part of such an attempt.

Table 4.14   System Simulation

Period	Arrivals from Tables 4.9 & 4.10	Times for Arrivals	Service Times from 4.13	Comments
1	3	15	20	Idle time till patient arrives
		30	15	Patient waits 5 minutes till patient 1 finished
		45	15	Patient waits 5 minutes till patient 2 finished
2	3	15	10	Idle time for 10 minutes after patient 3 departs.
		30	15	Idle time for 5 minutes after patient 4 departs

It is probably easier to visualise this on some form of
"time-line" - see Figure 4.2.

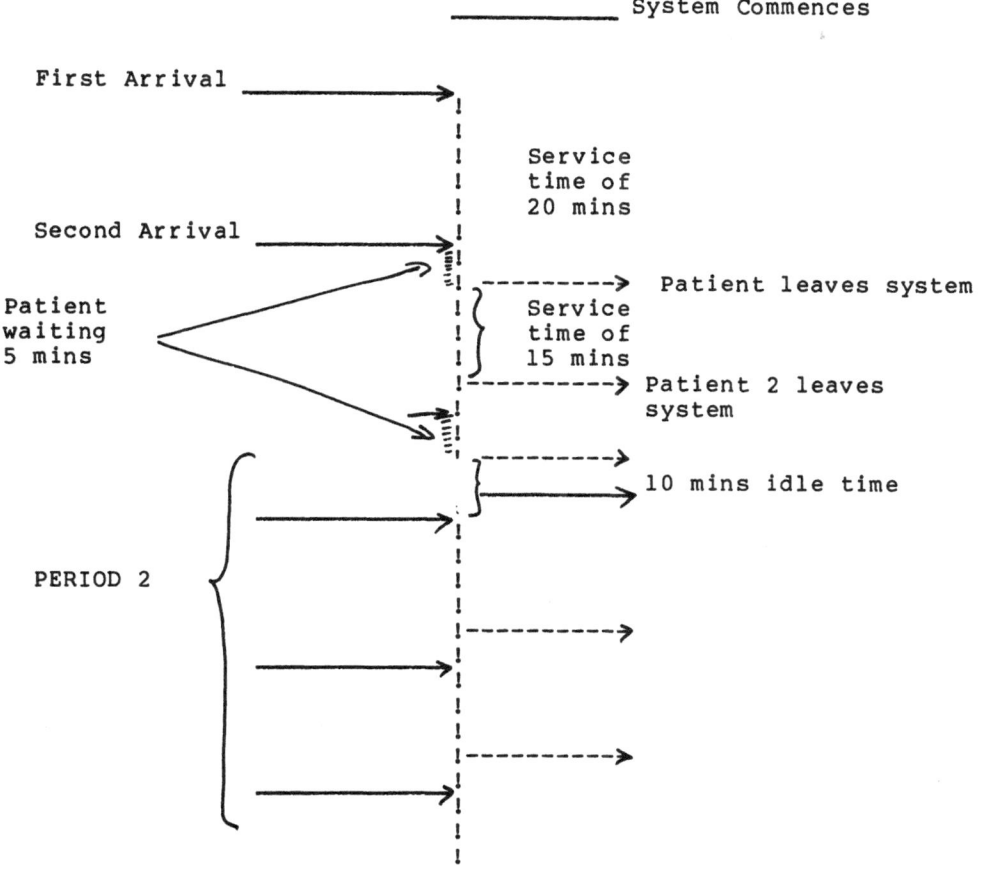

System Commences

Figure 4.2 The First 120 Minutes of the System

Table 4.14 and Figure 4.3 show that in period 1 the service facility is idle for the first 15 minutes and then an arrival takes place which is serviced for the next 20 minutes. However, after 30 minutes from the beginning of the period have elapsed, there is a further arrival which is not served immediately since the first customer is being served. Thus for 5 minutes a queue of 1 unit forms. Customer 1 departs at the end of the 35th minute and customer 2 is served from then for 15 minutes until minute 50. In the meantime customer 3 has arrived at the end of the 45th minute and forms a queue of one for 5 minutes. The customer is served for all ten remaining minutes of the period and since there is a 15 minute service time for this customer, service will carry over for 5 minutes of the 2nd period.

In period 2 there are 3 arrivals so the first takes place after 15 minutes. For the first 5 minutes the 3rd arrival of period 1 is being served, but for the next 10 minutes the facility is idle. The first customer of this period has a 10 minute service time and service is completed by the end of the 25th minute so there are 5 minutes idle time before customer 2 arrives at the 30th minute to be serviced for 15 minutes, at which time the 3rd customer arrives. By the end of the period the 3rd customer has been served for 15 minutes and still has 5 minutes to run. The experience in Periods 1 and 2 is summarised in Table 4.15.

Table 4.15   Queue Statistics - Periods 1 & 2

Period	Occasions of Idle Time	Idle Time	Queues	Queue Length	Queue Duration
1	1	15	2	1	5
				1	5
2	2	10 5	0		

The simulation of the other time periods proceeds in a similar manner. For period 3 the first 5 minutes are occupied by the carryover from period 2 and the facility is idle for the next 10 minutes. Service of the 3 arrivals (15 minutes service time each) takes place continuously over the remaining 43 minutes of the hour.

In period 4 there are no arrivals and with no carryover the service facility remains idle for the whole 60 minutes.

There are no arrivals in period 5. For period 6, since there are two arrivals the first is assumed to take place after 20 minutes (of idle time); 20 minutes of service time is required immediately after which the 2nd customer arrives requiring 5 minutes service time. For the remaining 15 minutes of the hour the facilities are idle.

In period 7 the facility is idle for the first 20 minutes and 2 services of 20 minutes each take up the rest of the hour.

Period 8. There is a period of 15 minutes idle time at the beginning of the period and 2 further idle times of 5 minutes with no queues forming.

Period 9. 15 minutes idle time followed by 15 minutes service and an arrival which requires 20 minutes. The 3rd customer therefore forms a queue for 5 minutes before being serviced at the end of the 50th minute. This customer still requires an addition 5 minutes at the end of the period.

In period 10 the first 5 minutes are taken up with carryover service. For a four customer arrival tour, the first arrival takes place after 12 minutes so 7 minutes of idle time are present. The first customer is serviced for 15 minutes until the end of the 27th minute; meanwhile the 2nd customer has arrived and waited for 3 minutes.

The 2nd customer requires 20 minutes service until the end of the 47th minute. In the meantime the 3rd customer has been waiting for 11 minutes. Customer 3 then takes up the remaining 13 minutes of the hour and has 2 minutes remaining. Meanwhile, customer 4 has been waiting in a queue of 1 for 12 minutes.

In period 11, customer 3 of the previous period is served for 2 minutes whilst customer 4 from the previous period waits in the queue and then is served for the next 10 minutes. The facility is idle for 3 minutes until customer 1 arrives for a 20 minute service. Customer 2 waits in a queue for 5 minutes and is serviced for 20 minutes to the end of the 55th minute. Customer 3 has had a 10 minute wait and has 15 minutes of his or her service time remaining at the end of the period. The process continues for the remaining periods of the simulation. The results are summarised in Table 4.16.

Table 4.16   Queue Statistics

Period	Occasions of Idle Time	Idle Time	Queues	Queue Length	Duration in minutes
1	1	15	2	1 1	5 5
2	2	10 5	0	-	-
3	1	10	0	-	-
4	1	60	0	-	-
5	1	60	0	-	-
6	2	20 15	0	-	-
7	1	20	0	-	-
8	3	15 5 5	0	-	-
9	1	15	1	1	1
10	1	7	3	-	3 11 12
11	1	3 — 265	3		2 5 10 58

For the 11 periods above statistics can be generated concerning

(i)   Idle Time

    (a)   Total Idle Time = 265 minutes

(b)   % of Idle Time $= \dfrac{\text{Total Idle Time}}{\text{Total Time Available}} \times \dfrac{100}{1}$

$= \dfrac{265}{11 \times 60} \times \dfrac{100}{1}$

$= \dfrac{26500}{660}$

$= 40.15\%$

(ii) Queues

(a)   Queues are present for 58 minutes

(b)   Average waiting time $= \dfrac{\text{Duration of Queues}}{\text{No. of Arrivals}}$

$= \dfrac{58}{26}$

$= 2.23$ minutes

(c)   Estimate of probability of obtaining a queue of

length 1 $= \dfrac{\text{Duration of queues}}{\text{Total Time Available}}$

$= \dfrac{58}{11 \times 60}$

$= \dfrac{58}{660}$

$= .087$

Note that queues of more than one customer do not occur during the first 11 periods. The results are, of course, simply designed to illustrate the process of obtaining the information about the characteristics of the system. A much larger number of periods would be required in practice to obtain meaningful results. It is evident that performing the simulation by hand for a reasonable number of periods (over 400 would probably be required to achieve stable results) is a very time consuming and tedious process. However, a computer may be readily programmed to perform the required simulation, and the results for a simulation of several thousand periods may be obtained very quickly.

SOME OBSERVATIONS

It should be noted that simulation provides for a great deal of flexibility in solving operations research problems. In queuing problems, for example, it may be desirable to assume that the service rate is dependent on the size of the queue; or varies with the time of day, or the time which has elapsed since the system involving the queue commenced operations. It is not wholly realistic to assume, as most mathematical queuing models do, that the service rate is independent of all these considerations. Whilst modifications of these kinds to the simulation procedure may be readily introduced (by simply altering the probability distribution of service times at the appropriate periods), it may be very difficult or impossible to achieve the same effect using the direct mathematical approach.

APPLICATIONS

As simulation is a relatively simple process and it allows one to experiment with alternative strategies, it is often regarded as the most useful operations research technique available for health service problems. However, development of a simulation model is extremely expensive in terms of personnel and often unrealistic in terms of information requirements.

Nevertheless, a large range of applications of simulation have been reported. Stimson & Stimson (1972) report many examples of applications of simulation to admission and utilization systems. Many applications are also recorded in traditional queuing areas such as outpatient departments and patient scheduling generally. Wren (1974) reports a number of applications of simulation to health planning including, for example, that of Brooks & Beenhakker (1964) which applied simulation techniques to estimate the future bed needs of a community. Palmer (1975) has reviewed a number of simulation models used for testing national health policy, hospital utilization and other areas. Fries (1981) also reviews the use of simulation in the health system.

Unfortunately the complexity of the information gathering process has hindered the development of simulation models of hospitals and health service problem areas. Most models are highly specific to the particular system studied and it is not easy to transfer a simulation model from, say a 1,000 bed teaching hospital to a 100 bed country hospital. However a number of computer 'simulation languages' (such as SIMSCRIPT, SIMULA & GPSS) have been developed to facilitate the development of simulation models. Some of these languages are reviewed in Gordon (1978).

A number of special purpose packages have also been developed which simulate operating theatres, casualty or outpatient clinics and so on. An example of such a package is the CLINIC Simulation Model (available from the National Technical Information Service, Springfield, Virginia: PB262 229) which is a computerised simulation model of a hospital outpatient/emergency room service. It provides for both walk-in and appointment patients. A flow diagram of possible patient paths through the system is shown in Figure 4.3 The model allows for certain parameters to be specified by the user thus facilitating adaption to the user's own facility and also allowing simulation of alternative arrangements.

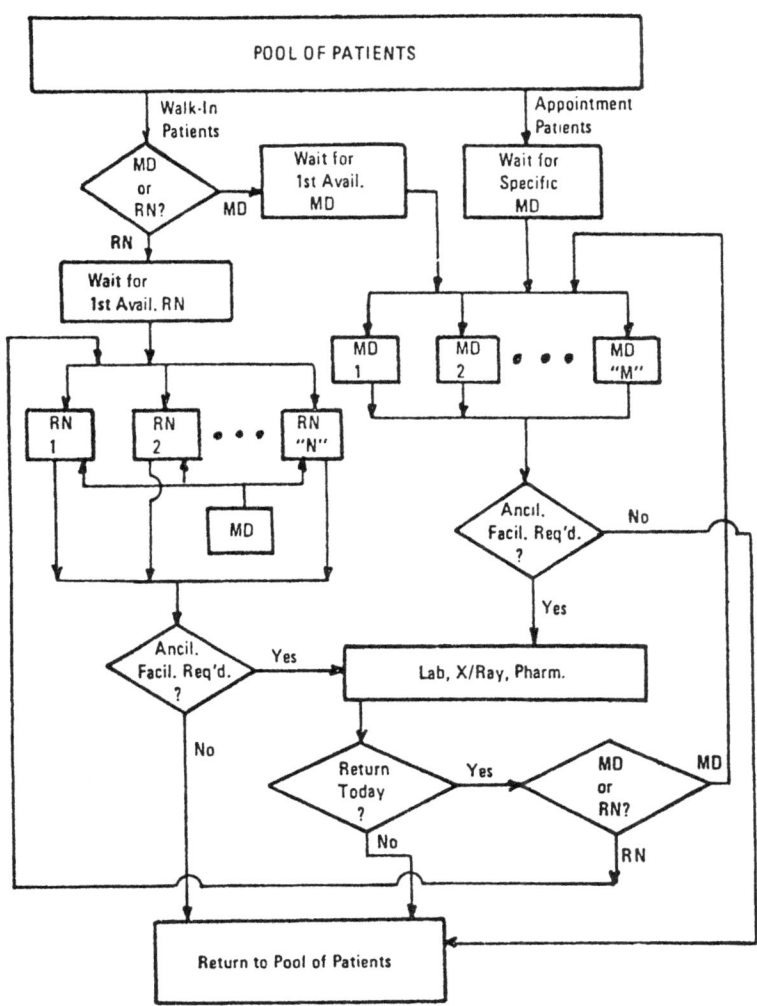

Figure 4.3   Schematic Patient Flow Diagram Indicating the Logic
              of the Simulation Program in the CLINIC Model

The model uses three types of data input:

1) Deterministic data which specify the clinic schedule (e.g. opening and closing times; when appointment patients have been scheduled; the time for coffee or meal breaks etc.).

2) Descriptive statistics which characterise the clinic being simulated (e.g. means and standard deviations of arrival rates and service times).

3) Data which specify the clinic arrangements (e.g. probability of walk in patient going to the Physician Clinic rather than the Nurse Practitioner Clinic).

The output from the CLINIC program includes statistics on percentage utilisation for physicians and nurses; waiting time for walk-in and appointment patients; total time in the system etc. Because of the format of the data input, it is relatively easy to test the effects of different numbers of staff, different expected number of patients and also more fundamental changes in system characteristics such as the ratio of nurse to physician contacts. A description of an application of the program may be found in Rising (1977).

CONCLUSION

The simulation technique we have described is sometimes referred to as the Monte Carlo method because the basis used to generate the simulations consists of a series of random trials analogous to playing a game of chance such as roulette. The technique may also be used to reproduce the properties of an inventory model containing probabilistic demand, or indeed of any mathematicaly or operations research model which processes some probabilistic element. It is, for example, possible to simulate the operations of an entire organization if comprehensive information is available about all elements making up the system.

Systems simulation thus provides a basis for carrying out fast, low cost experimentation. Experimentation by changing the actual system and measuring the effects is usually out of the question so that simulation becomes a most attractive alternative. Thus questions of how much will service be improved by adding additional channels, or what will happen if the priority rule governing the service to a queue (the queue discipline) is changed, may be resolved by using simulation.

Simulation, can assist at all stages of the decision making process of finding alternatives, of predicting the consequences of each and of choosing the most attractive set of consequences. It is not surprising, therefore, that following an extremely comprehensive review of uses of simulation in the health system, Valinsky (1975) reiterated Flagle's conclusion of a decade before that simulation,

"Of all the research techniques, it is the most comprehensible to the practitioner - the most difficult for the researcher to retreat to obscurantism, and it provides a bridge of communication between the two as well as a meeting ground for collaborative effort."

REFERENCES

Brooks, G.H. & Beenhakker, H.L. (1964) 'A New Technique for Production of Future Hospital Bed Needs', Hospital Management, pp.47-50, June.

Flagle, C.D. (1966) "Simulation Techniques Applicable to Public Health Administration" Proceedings on Simulation in Business & Public Health, First Annual Conference of American Statistical & Public Health Associations, New York.

Fries, B.E. (1981) Applications of Operations Research to Health Care Delivery Systems: A Complete Review of the Periodical Literature, (Lecture Notes in Medical Informatics No. 10), Springer Verlag.

Gaver, D.P. (1978) 'Simulation Theory' in Moder, J.J. & Elmaghraby, S.E. (eds.) Handbook of Operations Research: Foundations & Fundamentals, Van Nostrand Reinhold, pp.545-565.

Gordon, G. (1978) 'Simulation-Computation' in Moder, J.J. & Elmaghraby, S.E. (eds.) Handbook of Operations Research: Foundations & Fundamentals, Van Nostrand Reinhold, pp.566-585.

Hollingdale, S.H. (1978) 'Methods of Operational Analysis' in Lighthill, J. (ed.) Newer Uses of Mathematics, Penguin, pp.176-277.

Palmer, B.Z. (1975) 'Models in Planning & Operating Health Services' in Gass, S.I. & Sisson, R.L. (eds.) A Guide to Models in Governmental Planning & Operations, Sauger.

Rising, E.J. (1977) Ambulatory Care Systems Vol 1: Design for Improved Patient Flow, Lexington.

Stimson, D.H. & Stimson, R.H. (1972) Operations Research in Hospitals: Diagnosis and Prognosis, Hospital Research and Education Trust.

Valinsky, D. (1975) 'Simulation' in Shuman, L.J., Speas, R.D. & Young, J.P. (eds.) Operations Research in Health Care: A Critical Analysis, Johns Hopkins UP.

Wren, G. (1974) Modern Health Administration, Georgia U.P.

SIMULATION - SUMMARY

Simulation is a technique that can be used with any of the operations research problem types. It enables conclusions to be drawn when it is difficult to derive exact mathematical distributions.

A simulation of a system involves four main steps:-

1.   Derivation of the probability distribution of the various outcomes. For example, 3 arrivals (or units demanded) occurs with a probability of .2.

2.   Association of the various outcomes with certain numbers. Having determined the probability of an occurrence, that proportion of the numbers we are sampling from would be set aside to indicate that outcome.

3.   Using a table of random numbers (or a 'random number' generator), a sampling procedure is used to simulate a certain time period or series of events.

4.   Statistics are generated by averaging the results of the simulation.

5   ALLOCATION

It is often argued that the most difficult decisions that
management have to make are those concerning allocation of
resources: there are many things we would like to do but not
enough equipment, money or people to do them. Problems such as
these are known as allocation problems and operation research
techniques have been developed to assist solve these problems.
Allocation problems are concerned with assisting in the
allocation of scarce resources to meet competing demands in the
most effective way. There are two main subclassifications of
allocation problems: product mix and component mix.

(a)   Product Mix

It is obviously important to a manufacturer producing a number of
different items using limited equipment to allocate the available
facilities in the best possible way. Thus, for example, several
items could be produced each contributing to the overall profit,
assuming the manufacturer's aim is to maximise profit. The
allocation problem is to determine the optimum combination of
items (products). Like many other situations in operations
research, a solution of this kind of product mix problem is of a
short run nature since, in the long run, production facilities
could be expanded.

(b)   Component Mix or Blending problems

A manufacturer may also be faced with decisions concerning
blending of petrol, parts, fertilizers etc. The constituents are
available in limited quantities for certain prices. The problem
is to produce the least cost mixture which satisfies certain
minimum standards. The allocation problem is again to determine
the optimum combination of quantities.

All allocation problems have two basic elements:

    (1)   the objective one is working towards and
    (2)   the constraints that apply.

Typical allocation problems will appear as follows:-

    (a)   Establish a family planning program which maximises the
           number of births prevented annually subject to
           available finance and educational resources (an example
           of a product mix problem)

    (b)   Minimise total meal cost to patients ensuring that all
           patients receive sufficient calories and sufficient
           protein (an example of a component mix problem)

    (c)   Maximise the health of the community as provided by doctors and nurses bearing in mind that the more doctors that are trained, the fewer nurses and that doctors are more expensive than nurses.

    (d)   Maximise the care given to patients by ward staff (including a Charge Nurse, Registered Nurses, Student Nurses and Nursing Aides or Licensed Practical Nurses) subject to the fact that all have different rates of pay and some of them can't do certain activities.

Several techniques have been developed to solve these problems, more frequently, however, mathematicaly programming techniques are applied.

The simplest form of mathematical programming is known as <u>linear programming</u> which relates to the situation where the relationship between certain variables in the problem can be expressed in linear form (i.e. by straight lines).

<u>General Form</u>

The general algebraic format of both product mix and component mix examples is the same. As indicated above, all allocation problems involve a specified objective normally expressed as maximise P (or minimise P) where P is defined as, say, number of births prevented or total cost. In turn, this objective is elaborated and defined in terms of an <u>objective function</u>. Formulation of the objective function involves, as its name implies, expressing the objective as a function of relevant variables. In linear programming it will normally be in the form:

$$P = C_1 x_1 + C_2 x_2 + \ldots C_n x_n$$

Where the C_i are constants and the x_i are variables.

Let us assume our objective is to maximise the number of patients seen in a health care system (P). If the patients are basically of two kinds, hospital or health centre, we would attempt to maximise the following:

$$P = H + C$$
(H = number of patients seen in hospitals
C = number of patients seen in health centres)

We may place differing weights on the two variables to reflect differing policies. For example, we could regard a visit to a health centre as twice as useful as a visit to a hospital i.e. two hospital patients count the same as one health centre patient. We would then attempt to:

$$\text{maximise } P' = 2H + C$$

The <u>constraints</u> will be formulated as an algebraic expression being <u>less than</u>, less than or equal to, greater than or greater than or equal to a constant i.e. they will be of the form:

$$a_1 \; x_1 + a_2 \; x_2 + \ldots\ldots\ldots + a_n \; x_n \leqslant A$$

or $x_1 \geqslant 0$ etc.

Thus we may have a constraint that the total cost must be less than \$A or that a particular variable must not be negative e.g. there is no such thing as "negative doctors"!

In general a linear programming problem will be of the following form:

$$\text{Maximise } C = C_1 \; x_1 + C_2 \; x_2 + \ldots\ldots\ldots C_n \; x_n$$

$$\text{Subject to } a_{11} \; x_1 + a_{12} \; x_2 + \ldots\ldots\ldots + a_{1n} \; x_n \leqslant A_1$$

$$a_{21} \; x_1 + a_{22} \; x_2 + \ldots\ldots\ldots + a_{2n} \; x_n \leqslant A_2$$

$$a_{m1} \; x_1 + a_{m2} + \ldots\ldots\ldots + a_{mn} \; x_n \leqslant A_m$$

$$x_j \geqslant 0 \; \forall \; j \quad (\forall \text{ means "for all")}$$

Note that both the objective function and the constraints are linear. It is possible however to use linear programming for problems with a non linear objective function.

Linear programming problems can be solved graphically or by using an algorithm called the simplex method. Clearly a graphical solution becomes difficult if more than two variables are involved so we shall initially restrict ourselves to consideration of the two variable case. In our discussion the general form of the linear programming problem will involve a linear equation as an objective function to be optimised and several constraints expressed as linear inequalities of two variables.

GRAPHICAL SOLUTION

As we are dealing with only two variables, these can be easily plotted on a graph. A linear equation will divide the cartesian plane into two parts:

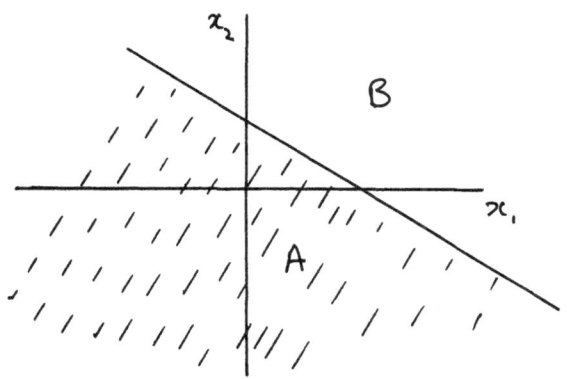

Figure 5.1

If the line has the equation $a_1x_1 + a_2x_2 = k$, (k any constant) one side of the line will include all the points which satisfy the inequation $a_1x_1+a_2x_2 > k$ and the other side $a_1x_1+ a_2x_2 < k$. (One can quickly determine which side is which by testing the origin (0,0): the expression is simple to evaluate $a_10+a_20 = 0$ and hence we can easily see if k is greater than or less than 0. Having determined which side the origin lies on, all other points follow.) Given an objective function and a set of constraints expressed as inequations, the graphical solution of linear programming problems is relatively straightforward.

First, we graph the equations from which the constraints are derived and shade in the appropriate areas to represent the inequations. There will normally be a small space common to all inequations i.e. a number of points which satisfy all the constraints (inequations). Obviously, the solution lies within this space and so it is called the <u>solution space</u>. (It is sometimes called the set of feasible solutions.) It can be shown that the optimal value (or values) will lie at one of the vertices of the solution space or along one of the boundaries.

There are two ways of proceeding to the second step, evaluation of which of the points in the solution space is the optimal solution. One approach is to substitute the coordinates of each of the vertices into the objective function and the one which yields the maximum (or in a minimising problem, the minimum) value is thus the optimal point. Where two of the vertices yield equal optimal values, then those two points, and the straight line joining them, are optimal. The second approach is to draw a set of parallel lines representing different levels of the objective function on the graph. The coordinates of the optimising vertex yield the solution to our initial problem.

Often the most difficult part of a linear programming problem is identifying the objective function, selecting the variables and formulating the constraint equations. The following two examples of that process (including the final step of graphing the solution) provide a step by step account of the processes.

<u>Example 5.1: A product mix problem</u>

Grundy and Reinke (1973) discuss a linear programming model for planning a community health programme. The problem is formulated as follows:-

> "Suppose, for example, that a family planning programme
> is intended to maximize the number of births prevented
> annually, and that four woman-years of IUD protection
> or two woman-years of oral contraception are required
> to prevent one birth. What is the ideal contraceptive
> mix to be sought in order to maximize births
> prevented?"

In this case the objective is clearly stated and can be expressed in linear form: maximize the number of births prevented. Information on relative weights in the objective function is also provided. In this case if one wants to prevent 1,000 births annually one can either have 4,000 women using IUD's (since there is one birth prevented for every four woman-years of IUD use) or of these (i.e. if 2,000 women use IUD's and 1,000 women use oral contraceptives 1,000 births will still be prevented).

Similarly if one wants to prevent 500 births per annum, one can have either 2,000 women using IUD's or 1,000 women using oral contraceptives or any linear combination of these.

The number of births prevented (B) can be expressed as a linear combination of the number of IUD users (D) and the number of users of oral contraceptives (P). As four woman-years of IUD protetion prevents one birth, algebraically one woman-year of IUD protection prevents 1/4 birth. Hence the weight for IUD protection is .25. Similarly, the weight for use of oral contraceptives is .5. The equation relating IUD protection and oral contraceptive use is:

$$B = .25 D + .5P$$

and the objective function becomes

$$\text{Maximize } B = .25 D + .5P$$

This can be portrayed graphically as follows:

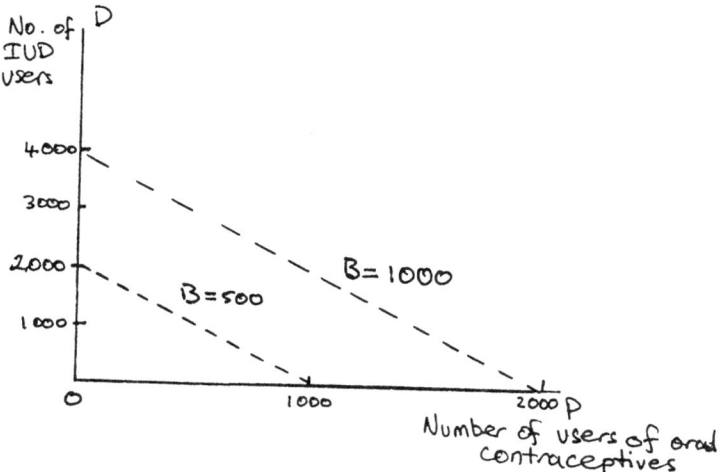

Figure 5.2

The parallel lines show different numbers of births prevented per
annum and the further one moves from the origin (0,0), the more
births are prevented. The parallel lines are sometimes called
"frontiers".

Of course, no constraints are shown on the diagram but in
practice constraints on human resources, availability of IUD's
and availability of finance may apply. Grundy and Reinke add:

> "Consider possible manpower limitations first. Let us
> suppose that our family planning clinic has only four
> workers each available for 2,000 hours per year; and
> that they require three hours of activity for each
> oral contraceptor and two hours for each IUD user."

Thus the human resource constraint refers to the fact that a
total of 8,000 hours (4 workers, 2000 hours each) are available
to implement the scheme in any one year and that each user of
oral contraceptives requires three hours and each IUD user
requires two hours. If we were to have no IUD users, we could
have 2666 users of oral contraceptives since we have 8,000 hours
available and each oral contraceptor requires three hours
(8,000/3 = 2,666). Similarly if we have no users of oral
contraceptives we could have 4,000 users of IUDs. But in fact
our total number of hours can be made up of any linear
combination of these figures. For each IUD user two hours of
worker time is required and for each user of oral contraceptives
three hours is required, the combined total of these hours must
be less than the 8,000 hours available. The human resource
constraint may be expressed mathematically as follows:-

$$8,000 \ngtr 2 D + 3 P$$
$$\text{or } 2D + 3 P \leqslant 8,000$$

and since $2(0) + 3(0) \leqslant 8,000$, the origin is a feasible solution.
The inequation can be graphed as follows:

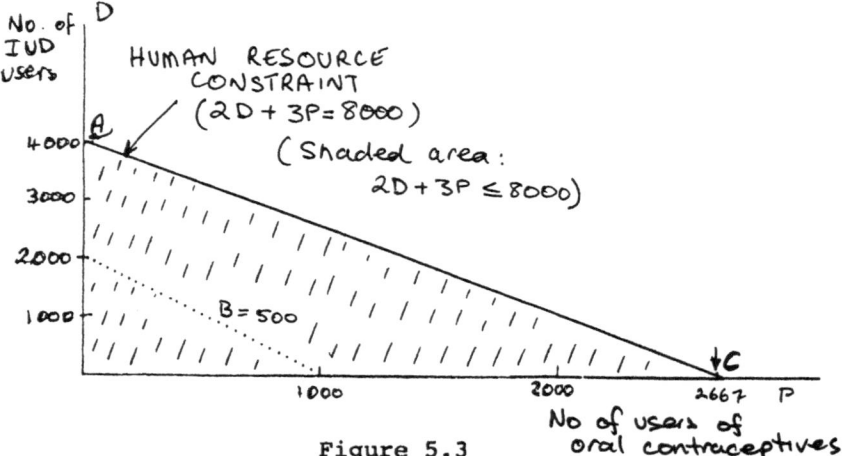

Figure 5.3

Given this one constraint, any point in the triangle AOC is a
feasible solution. The optimum solution, however, is one which
maximizes the births prevented i.e. that point within the
triangle AOC which is on the parallel line (B frontier) furthest

from the origin.   As the point C is on the highest B frontier
(B=2,667), if there were no further constraints C would be the
optimum solution.   Grundy & Reinke, however, go on to say:-

> "Now let us introduce a financial constraint. We shall
> suppose that each womn year of oral protection costs
> $80, each woman year of IUD protection costs $15 and
> the programme has a total budget of $100,000."

This financial constraint can be expressed mathematically as:
$$15D + 80P \leq 100,000$$
and can be included on the diagram as follows:-

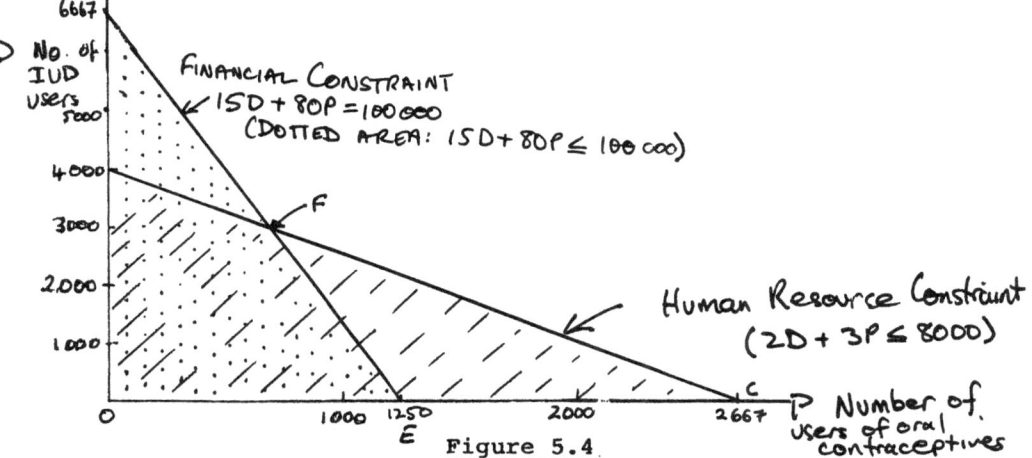

Figure 5.4

As we have now included all the constraints on the graph we can
now determine the optimum combination of methods.   The simplest
way of doing this is to return to the set of parallel lines that
represent the objective function (see Figure 5.2).   Now it will
be recalled that the further away from (0,0) the parallel line
is, the more births are prevented.   We can draw a series of
parallel lines on   Figure 5.4 to represent different numbers of
births prevented (see Figure 5.5)

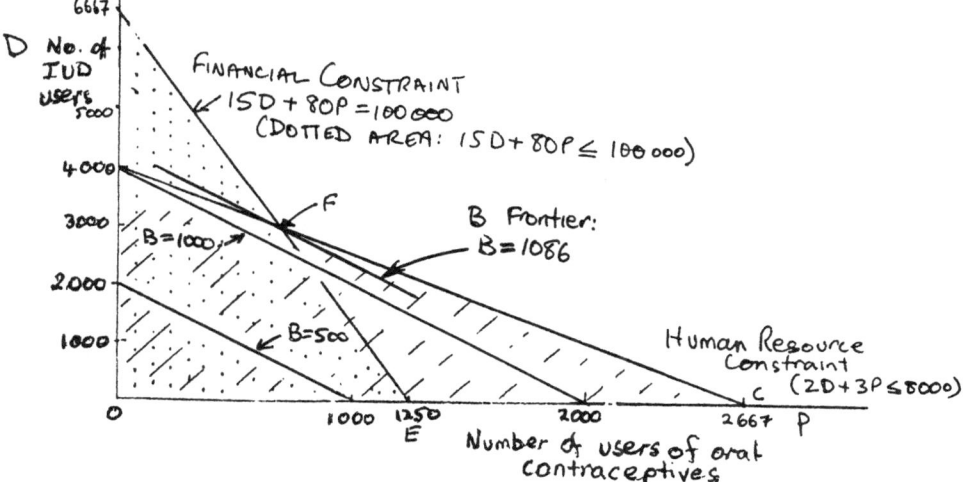

Figure 5.5

It can be seen that point F is on the parallel line furthest from (0,0). If we had drawn our graph accurately, we could determine the optimum combination of oral contraceptors and IUD users by reading off the coordinates of point F. It turns out that these are (695,2956) and thus we should plan to have 695 women using oral contraceptives and 2956 using IUDs. Substituting these figures in our original objective function (.25D + .5P), we see that 1085 births will be prevented (.25 x 2956 + .5 x 695 = 1086).

It will be recalled that the optimum solution in a linear programming problem is always one of the vertices or a line joining them (when the objective function is linear). We can therefore also determine the optimum solution by evaluating he value of the objective function at each of the vertices of the solution space AOEF. We can determine the actual value of these points either by reading off from the graph or by calculating the points of intersection using simultaneous equations.

```
In this case at 0,  B = .25D + .5P becomes
                    B = .25(0) + .5(0) = 0
at A,               B = .25 (4000) + .5(0) = 1000
at E,               B = .25(0) + .5 (1250) =   625
from the graph, F is the point (695,2956)
and                 B = .25 (2956) + .5(695)
                      = 1086
```

Again, we reach the same optimal solution, namely to have 695 women using oral contraceptives and 2956 women using IUDs, since it is at this point that .25D + .5P is maximised.

A cautionary word

The linear programming solution is optimal in a technical sense, and the values underlying the choice of constraints, for example, may not be the same as those of the women (and men) affected.

As in all operations research examples, the mathematical techniques are supplements to or parts of the decision making process - they do not provide the whole answer.

Example 5.2: A component mix problem

A typical component mix type problem in the health services is the diet problem. The objective is to ensure that a patient's diet includes maximum quantities of certain nutrients but is provided at minimum cost.

Let us consider two foodstuffs, wholemeal bread and cheddar cheese, each containing three nutrients: kilojoules, grams of protein and micrograms of thiamine. From food composition tables, we know that each kilogram of wholemeal bread contains 9,500 kilojoules, 100 grams protein an 2,500 micrograms of thiamine. For cheddar cheese the corresponding values are 17,000 kilojoules, 250 grams, and 350 micrograms.

The dietitians have advised that each patient must have at least 10,000 kilojoules per day, at least 70 grams of protein, and at least 1,000 micrograms of thiamine. The catering manager has advised that the price of wholemeal bread is 120¢ per kilo and

cheddar cheese is obtained at 350¢ per kilo. Our objective is to
determine the least cost diet of the two foodstuffs which
satisfies the nutritional requirements.

Let T = total cost
   B = kilograms of bread consumed
   C = kilograms of cheese consumed

As each kilo of bread costs 120¢ and each kilo of cheese, 350¢
total cost will simply be the sum of the product of price and
quantity for each item.

Algebraically we wish to
minimise T = 120B + 350C

subject to constraints concerning kilojoules, grams of protein,
and micrograms of thiamine.

Now, for each kilo of bread consumed, a patient obtains 9,500
kilojoules and for each kilo of cheese consumed a patient
obtains 17,000 kilojoules. Since a minimum of 10,000 kilojoules
is to be consumed the constraint concerning kilojoules can be
expressed as:

$9,500B + 17,000C \geqslant 10,000$
i.e., $19B + 34C \geqslant 20$

Similarly from the data concerning the number of grams of protein
and micrograms of thiamine in a kilo of each of the substances we
can deduce the other constraints.

Protein constraint:

$100B + 250C \geqslant 70$

i.e., $10B + 25C \geqslant 7$

Thiamine constraint:

$2,500B + 350C \geqslant 1,000$

i.e., $50B + 7C \geqslant 20$

The problem can now be expressed as minimising

$\qquad T = 120B + 350C$

subject to $19B + 34C \geqslant 20$ (kilojoules constraint)
$\qquad\quad 10B + 25C \geqslant 7$ (protein constraint)
$\qquad\quad 50B + 7C \geqslant 20$ (thiamine constraint)

As there are only two variables, this can be plotted graphically,
this time with three constraint lines (see Figure 5.6). The
shaded area shows the points which satisfy all three constraints.
Note that the protein and kilojoule constraint lines do not
intersect and that all points which satisfy the kilojoule
constraint also satisfy the protein constraint. The protein
constraint is said to be non-binding.

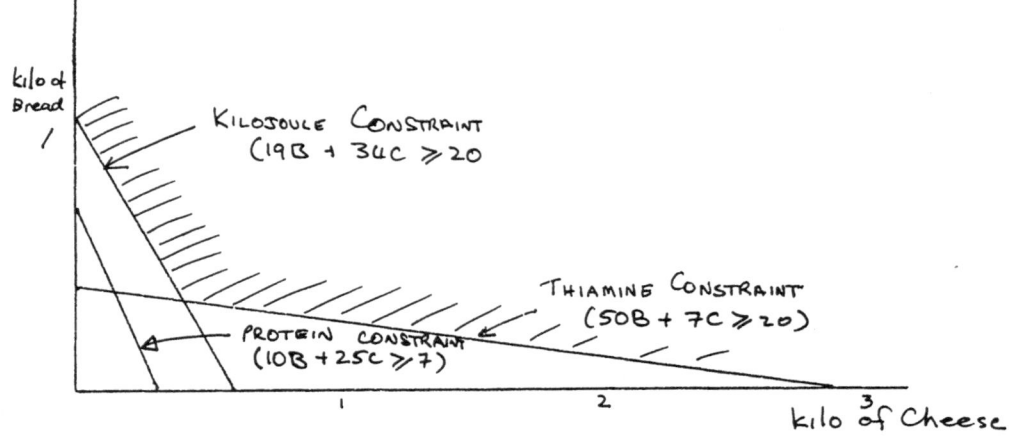

Figure 5.6

After including parallel lines representing the various levels of
total cost, we can read off the least cost composition which
meets the nutritional requirements (see Figure 5.6).

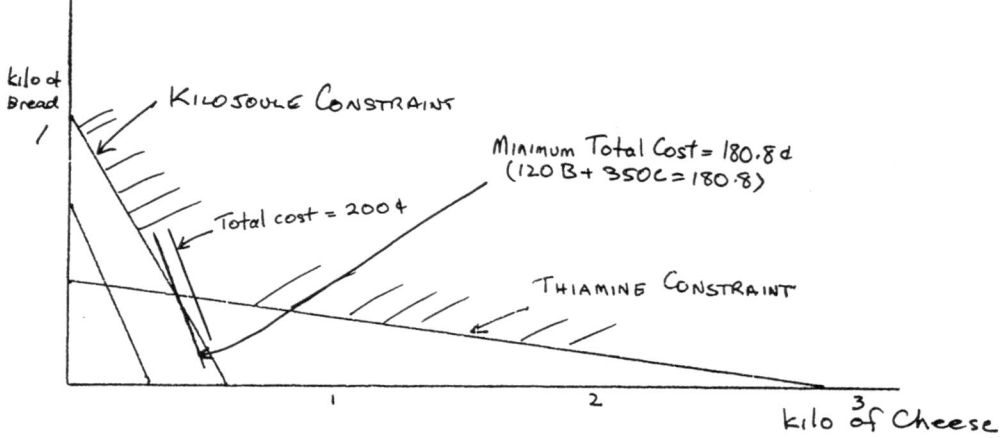

Figure 5.7

From the graph we can see that the optimum diet consists of 0.34
kilo of bread and 0.4 kilo of cheese and the·cost is 180.8¢. It
is easily verified that this diet satisfies the nutritional
requirements. (Solving the two binding constraints
simultaneously yields an optimal solution of .3446 kilo of bread
and .954 kilo of cheese at a cost of 179.7¢.)

ALGEBRAIC SOLUTIONS

Except in a few special cases there is no direct mathematical method of solving linear programming problems. The difficulty is a consequence of the fact that there are an infinite number of possible values of the variables which will satisfy the inequality constraints. Amongst all these feasible solutions there is normally only one solution, the optimum feasible solution, which yields a minimum or maximum value for the objective function. It is generally the case that the only way in which the optimum solution may be identified is by a trial and error procedure, the most commonly used being known as the simplex method. The details of the method are somewhat complex and will not be discussed here, it is sufficient to note that this is a systematic and efficient procedure for generating feasible solutions each one superior to its predecessor. A fairly rapid approach is made to finding the optimum feasible solution, sometimes known as the basic solution.

Slack Variables

The constraint inequalities can be converted to equations by use of slack and artificial variables. For example, the inequality

$$2D + 3P \leqslant 8000$$

can be converted to an equation by the addition of a slack variable, S_1 (which takes up 'the slack'):

$$2D + 3P + S_1 = 8000$$

Sometimes it is useful to keep slack variables positive and hence artificial variables are introduced when necessary, for example the inequality

$$B + 2C \geqslant 3$$

requires a negative number on the left hand side to convert it into an equation, this negative number is formed by a positive slack variable and an artificial variable.

$$B + 2C + S_2 + A_2 = 3$$

The linear programming problem given in 5.1 thus becomes

$$\text{maximise} \quad .25D + .5P$$
$$\text{subject to} \quad 2D + 3P + S_1 = 8000$$
$$15D + 80P + S_2 = 100000$$

This can be solved using the simplex method the result, of course, being the same as before (D = 2956.52, P = 695.65 objective function at 1086.95).

Duality

Complex linear programming problems can be solved by use of principles of duality. Every linear programming problem has a dual formed by a reversal process, for example, the problem given in 5.1 was expressed in primal form:

$$\text{Maximise } .25D + .5P$$
$$\text{Subject to } 2D + 3P \leqslant 8000$$
$$15D + 80P \leqslant 100000$$

The dual of this is:

$$\text{Minimise } 8000M + 100000\ S$$
$$\text{Subject to } 2M + 15S \geqslant .25$$
$$3M + 80S \geqslant .5$$

This is roughly analogous to turning the problem on its side and reversing the signs.

The problem can be solved graphically yielding an optimal solution of $M = .1086$ and $S = .00217$, the objective function then being 1086.956.

It is important to note that the value of the objective function in the dual is exactly the same as the value of the objective function in the primal solution. Use of the dual formulation allows conversion of a problem with many variables but only two constraints, into a problem with many constraints but only two variables. There are a number of similar corresponding results discussed fully in most texts on operations research.

The Simplex Solution

The simplex solution also provides information relating to the slack variables, which indicates how the objective function would change if there were changes in the slack variable. As the solution is already optimal, increasing one slack variable must imply a move to a non optimal solution with D & P at different values; this would yield a reduction in our objective function, the extent of the reduction being determined from our simplex solution. In example 5.1 an increase in S_1 of 1 unit would yield a reduction in the objective function of $.1086$ units. Similarly an increase in S_2 of 1 unit would yield a reduction in the objective function of $.00217$ units. It can be shown that these are the activity levels of the variables in the dual problem. These values have an even more important interpretation. Let us assume that our original human resource constraint in example 5.1 was 8001 hours instead of 8000 hours, the objective function could now be maximised at exactly $.1086$ units greater (exactly the same amount as it would have been decreased if we had increased the slack or reduced the capacity). Such an interpretation has a direct correspondence with marginal value in economics and the $.1086$ is the marginal value of labour. This value is often known as the <u>shadow price.</u> Although our examples primarily have the objective function in non-price terms, we will use the term 'shadow price' to maintain consistency with other literature. A discussion of the uses of shadow prices will be undertaken in the section on applications of linear programming.

Computer Solutions

Computer programs are now readily available which utilize the simplex procedure to yield a solution even when more than a hundred variables and constraint inequalities are present in the problem. One such program or package is the Multi-purpose Optimization System developed at the Vogelback Computing Centre at Northwestern University, Chicago. This package uses simple english in a logical sequence to solve the problem. For example the input for the family planning example (5.1) would be as follows:-

```
Regular
Variables
D P
Maximize
.25D +. 5P
Constraints
2D + 3P = 8000
15D + 80P = 100000
Optimize
```

The output would include the following table:

Summary of Results

Variable No.	Variable Name	Basic Non-Basic	Activity Level	Opportunity Cost	Row No.
1	D	B	2956.5217391	----	
2	P	B	695.6521739	----	
3	--Slack	NB	---	.1086957	(1)
4	--Slack	NB	---	.0021739	(2)

Maximum value of the objective function = 1086.956522

It can be seen that the shadow prices yielded from the slack variables are displayed.

APPLICATIONS TO HEALTH ADMINISTRATION

a) Diet problem

The diet problem used in example 5.2 is a typical example of linear programming in health services. Balintfy and Nebel (1966) introduced a menu planning system using linear programming methods in which a computer was used to assist dietitians in preparing cost-minimising menus subject to certain minimal levels for several constraints. The results showed that menus planned without computer assistance had a higher (but more varying) level of nutritional satisfaction than menus planned with computer assistance (nevertheless, both menus were regarded as being acceptable to patients). The menus prepared using the linear programming model satisfied the nutritional requirements and were cheaper than the ones prepared by the dietitians.

Since this early application, a number of computerised linear programming based models have been developed to take account of the special diets hospital patients require (e.g. Hoover et al, 1982).

b) Hospital Management

Griffith (1972) reviews a number of applications of linear programming to hospital management. Perhaps the most ambitious is that of Dowling (1970, 1975), who argued that the activity, objectives and constraints of a hospital can be formulated using linear programming. Conceptually the model is simple and Dowling provided an example using two variables (the numbers of "medical" and "surgical" patients) with constraints relating to nursing hours, operating rooms, laboratory tests etc. Usage by medical and surgical patients of each of the constraint services is also calculated. Formulation of the objective function presents problems for the model builder and may introduce concepts of profit (or excess of revenue over costs for the different classification of patients) or relate to additional community costs if patients are not treated. The simplest objective function is to maximise the total number of patients treated. The solution of the allocation problem would then reveal the "optimum" numbers of medical and surgical patients.

In his simple example Dowling (1975, pp. 30-35) used an objective function of maximising the number of medical and surgical patients. The constraints related to the available facilities within the hospital and utilisation of these by patients in the two categories. Table 5.1 shows utilisation of the constraints and the capacity available.

TABLE 5.1   SIMPLE HOSPITAL UTILISATION AND CONSTRAINTS TABLE

| | UTILISATION | | CAPACITY |
INPUTS	MEDICAL PATIENTS	SURGICAL PATIENTS	AVAILABLE (PER ANNUM)
Nursing Days	9	7	73 000
Operations	–	1	6 000
Laboratory Tests	15	12	105 000
Physiotherapy Treatments	1	2	13 500
X-Ray Procedures	4	2	23 400

Thus, for example, each medical patient in this example uses 9 days of nursing care per 15 laboratory tests etc.

The problem is formulated:

$$\text{Maximize} \quad M + S$$

(where M = number of medical patients treated per year;
S = number of surgical patients treated per year.)

$$\text{subject to} \quad 9M + 7S \leqslant 73\ 000 \quad \text{(nursing days constraint)}$$

$$S \leqslant 6\ 000 \quad \text{(operations constraint)}$$

$$15M + 12S \leqslant 105\ 000 \quad \text{(lab. tests constraint)}$$

$$M + 2S \leqslant 13\ 500 \quad \text{(physiotherapy constraint)}$$

$$4M + 2S \leqslant 23\ 400 \quad \text{(x-ray constraint)}$$

This may be solved graphically (see Diagram 5.7 taken from Dowling, 1975).

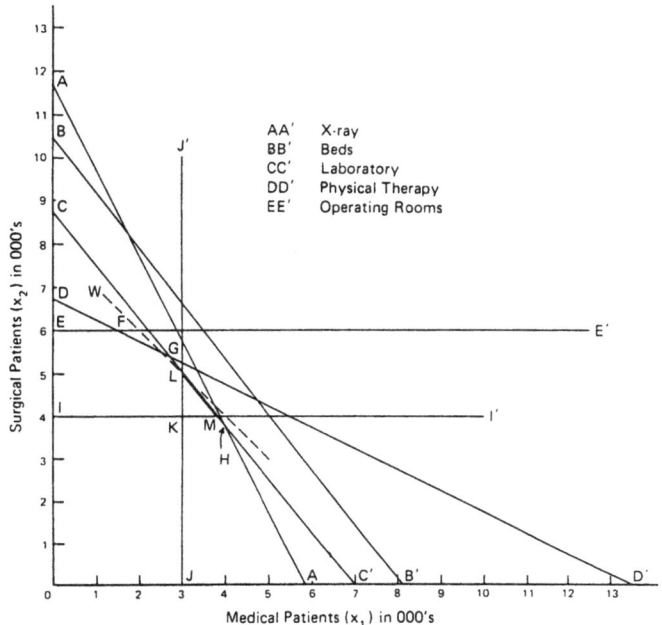

Figure 5.8 HOSPITAL PRODUCTION MODEL

It can be calculated that the optimal solution is to treat 2667 medical patients and 5417 surgical patients, yielding a total of 8084 patients treated per annum. (The parallel lines in Diagram 5.7 are the family of objective function lines.)

Obviously a hospital is much more complex than this. In the model Dowling developed (1975, p684) he used 55 variables representing 55 different diagnostic categories listed in Table 5.2.

A total of 14 constraints were used: nursing days; days in intensive care; units of blood consumed; EKG (ECG) examinations; Laboratory tests; IPPB services (intermittant positive pressure breathing services - a form of respirator services); hours of oxygen; IV fluids; prescriptions; x-ray films; number of deliveries; anaesthesia hours; operating room hours and recovery room hours. Data on utilisation of these inputs were obtained from PAS/MAP data compiled by study hospitals into a 55 x 14 matrix showing utilisation by each category (analogous to table 5.1). The capacity constraints were determined and an optimal solution for the number of patients in each category developed. The model also allowed the hospital to identify the binding constraints and the effect of increasing capacity on its objectives.

TABLE 5.2   DIAGNOSTIC CATEGORIES USED IN THE HOSPITAL PRODUCTION
             MODEL.

Pediatric Service

1. Infective
2. Eye
3. Ear
4. Acute upper respiratory
    infection
5. Pneumonia and bronchitis
6. Hypertrophy of tonsils
    and adenoids
7. Appendix
8. Hernia
9. Other gastrointestinal
10. Genitourinary
11. Fractures
12. Other trauma
13. Adverse effects
14. Other pediatric

Medical-Surgical Service

15. Infective
16. Malignant neoplasms
17. Other neoplasms
18. Diabetes mellitus
19. Endocrine, nutritional,
    and metabolic
20. Hematologic
21. Other nervous system
22. Eye
23. Ear
24. Hypertension
25. Acute myocardial
    infarction
26. Other heart
27. Cerebrovascular
28. Acute upper respiratory
    infection

30. Pneumonia and bronchitis
31. Hypertrophy of tonsils
    and adenoids
32. Other respiratory
33. Dental
34. Peptic ulser
35. Other upper
    pastrointestinal
36. Appndix
37. Hernia
38. Cholecystitis and
    calculus
39. Other gastrointestinal
40. Genitourinary
41. Breast
42. Female genital
43. Skin
44. Musculosketal
45. Congenital anomalies
46. Symptoms, Signs
47. Fractures
49. Adverse effects
50. Special conditions

Psychiatric Services

51. Mental

Obstetric Service

52. Complications of
    pregnancy
54. Deliveries

Newborn Service

55. Newborn

c) Workforce (manpower) planning

Workforce planning has been a fruitful field for the application
of linear programming. Most workforce problems fall easily into
the objective - constraints model of allocation problems and data
relating to constraints and objectives are often easy to obtain.

As indicated earlier, many problems facing managers can be
modelled using linear or mathematical programming. Shuman &
Wolfe (1975) in their review of applications of mathematical
programming in the health field, have suggested it is the most
emphasised technique in academic operations research programs,
although it has not lived up to expectations. The discussions
below, however outline several useful areas of application of
mathematical or linear programming.

Morgan (1970) for example illustrates the use of linear
programming at a micro level. He analyses the promotion policy

of a large bureaucracy (specifically a United Kingdom civil service authority) as an allocation policy: the problem being to allocate various people to the jobs that are available. Constraints reflect the number of people eligible for promotion, the number of positions that will fall vacant, the age distribution of people in senior posts etc. Morgan notes that the objective function may vary but could include cost minimisation or minimising the average age of those below a senior grade. The choice of an objective function relates, of course, to the goals of the bureaucracy as specified by those developing the model.

Reinke (1971) formulates a problem for optimizing the provision of health care in the community. The objective function in this instance is to determine the optimum number of medical and nursing practitioners. An assumption is made that each doctor produces five service units for every one contributed by each nurse.

Constraints reflect the number of existing practitioners and constraints on money available for salaries and the availability of training facilities. As the constraints are linear, the allcation problem resolves into a simple product mix with four constraints.

Another staffing or workforce planning problem that faces administrators is determining the optimal mix of different levels or classes of health personnel, although these could easily be classified as examples of hospital management problems. Wolfe (1964) describes a linear programming procedure for determining the optimal mix of the various levels of nursing personnel. The objective function is one of cost minimisation, determined by a combination of labour costs and imputed costs to account for the intangible costs deriving from "quality" differences in the level of care given by the various categories of nursing personnel. Derivation of the constraints involved an assumption that staff could only work a full shift and hence a 'dummy' idle time variable was also required.

Rothstein (1973) expanded this "rostering" problem by viewing the rostering of housekeeping staff (porters, maids etc.) as an allocation problem. Here several inequations were formulated in terms of various combinations of "days off" (eg x_1 = number of Mon-Tuesday off pairs). The numbers of personnel required on each day were used as constraint equations and an objective function of maximising the number of consecutive days off for employees was formulated. The model was applied with these constraints and again with an additional constraint ensuring a minimum number of shifts with Saturday and Sunday as days off.

As nurses comprise such a large proportion of the hospital (or other health facility) workforce, a number of papers have been written using operations research (generally linear or mathematical programming) to assist in nurse staffing and allocation. A review of recent papers in this field is included in Bennett and Duckett (1981).

d)   Health Planning

A number of studies have used linear or mathematical programming techniques to study large scale health planning problems. Bodin et al (1972) for example, developed a model for financing mental health services in New York involving a quadratic objective function. The model included recognition of political constraints. Heiner et al (1981) also used a linear programming formulation of cost and capacity constraints to develop a resource allocation model for mental retardation services.

Allocation techniques have also been used in planning general hospital services. Kao & Tung (1981) and Ruth (1981) both used allocation models to determine appropriate mixes of categories of beds to meet regional hospital needs.

A comprehensive health planning problem addressed by Feldstein et al (1973) using mathematical programming was the choice of an optimum strategy for tuberculosis control. The objective function was one of maximising the benefits which accrue subject to certain demographic and epidemiological constraints. The derivation of the objective function, like all measures of the benefits of health programs, proved difficult but a function combining the amount of benefit, the number of people benefiting and the "social value" of the benefit was eventually determined for each possible service type. Constraints were expressed in terms of requirements for money, skilled personnel and beds and in terms of population coverage for the entire program (broken down into specified proportions of several discrete population groups). The model deroves the optimal mix of treatment and programs for the various groups (eg. direct BCG vaccination or primary case finding and domicilliary treatment etc.)

System-wide applications of allocation models have also been undertaken. West (1981) for example, used a linear programming formulation in his discussion of the United Kingdom attempts to reallocate health resources between regions. Aspden et al (1981) also used an allocation model for allocation of health resources in Czechoslavakia.

The Use of Shadow Prices

When we introduced the concept of a 'shadow price' we drew attention to the parallel to the economic concept of marginal value. The shadow price has an important application in the derivation of marginal values in situations where the objective function is measured in dollar terms. In the examples given, the marginal value of personnel would indicate how much the manager should be prepared to pay for additional staff if available. As much of the health sector (and in fact many areas of government operation) is characterised by imperfect markets and hence possibly inappropriate market valuations of resources, the 'shadow' price can be used as a surrogate for the market price when making resource allocation decisions.

Another important use of shadow prices has been to improve the workings of decentralised decision making. In this instance the shadow price (or accounting price) can be viewed as the contribution of a particular resource to the objective function or 'profit'. This interpretation would allow a centralised organisation to devolve responsibility onto local managers and allow them to consume as much of any resource desired but each decentralised unit will be charged the shadow price for resources consumed. Because of the nature of the linear programming formulation this will ensure that each decentralised unit will, in fact, be working towards maximising the 'profit' of the overall organisation. Such a method has been adapted for use in centrally planned economies and large private enterprises to help attain the benefits of central planning without foregoing the loss of individual initiative.

As indicated above, the Dowling study reveals information about shadow prices in the study hospital. An examination of the binding constraints and the associated shadow prices reveals the extent to which hospital output (i.e. number of patients treated in the relevant diagnostic category) can be increased following changes in the capacity for the binding constraints.

Similarly it shows the constraints which are not binding and thus where other outputs (e.g. outpatient services) can be expanded without requiring expansion in hospital facilities. As an interesting aside Dowling compares actual operating levels with optimal operating levels to get a measure of efficiency of hospital production.

CONCLUSION

Linear and mathematical programming models can assist in numerous ways in the allocation of limited resources to achieve certain objectives. Their use implies that objectives have been specified and quantified and constraints are recognized and also quantified. This quantification process may be extremely difficult. However recognition of objectives and constraints, whether or not the next step of quantification and inclusion in a mathematical model is undertaken, is of great value to managers and planners.

Indeed allocation problems may be the most important types of problems facing health administrators and planners in future and the increasing importance of problems of allocating resources in the health sector will cause greater attention to be paid to rational methods of solution.

REFERENCES

Aspden, P. Mayhew, L. & Rusnak, M. (1981) "DRAM: A Model of Health Care Resource Allocation in Czechoslavakia" Omega. The International Journal of Management Science Vol. 9, No. 5, pp.509-518.

Balintly, J.L. & Nebel, E.C., (1966) "Experiments with Computer Assisted Menu Planning, Hospitals J.A.H.A., 40 (June 16) pp.88-96.

Bennett, T.R. & Duckett, S.J. (1981) "Operations Research & Nurse Staffing" International Journal of Biomedical Computing Vol. 12, pp.433-438.

Dowling, William L., (1970) "A Linear Programming Approach to the Analysis of Hospital Production", PhD thesis, U. of Michigan, Ann Arbor.

Dowling, William L., (1975) The Analysis of Hospital Production: A Linear Programming Approach, Heath.

Feldstein, M.S., Piot, M.A. & Sundaresan, T.L., (1973) Resource Allocation Model for Public Health Planning. A Case Study of Tuberculosis Control, WHO.

Griffith, J.R., (1972) Quantitative Techniques for Hospital Planning and Control, Heath Lexington.

Grundy, F. & Reinke, W., (1973) Health Practice Research and Formalized Managerial Methods, (Public Health Paper No. 51) WHO.

Heiner, K., Wallace, W.A. & Young, K. (1981) "A Resource Allocation & Evaluation Model for Providing Services to the Mentally Retarded" Management Science, Vol. 27, No. 7, July, pp.769-784.

Hoover, L.W., Waller, A.L., Rastkar, A. & Johnson, V.A. (1982) "Development of an On-line Real-time Menu Management System" Journal of American Dietetic Association, Vol. 80, No. 1, January, pp.46-51.

Kao, E.P.C. & Tung, G.G. (1981) "Bed allocation in a public health care delivery system", Management Science Vol. 27, No. 5, May, pp.507-520.

Morgan, R.W., (1970) "Linear Programming in Manpower Planning" in Smith, A.R., (ed.) Some Statistical Techniques in Manpower Planning, (CAS Occasional Paper No. 15) HMSO.

Reinke, W.A., (1971) Health Planning: Qualitative Aspects and Quantitative Techniques, Johns Hopkins University.

Rothstein, M., (1973) "Hospital Manpower Shift Scheduling by Mathematical Programming", Health Services Research, Vol. 8, No. 1, Spring, pp.60-66.

Ruth, R.J. (1981) "A Mixed Integer Programming Model for Regional Planning of a Hospital Inpatient Service" Management Science Vol. 27, No. 5, May, pp.521-533.

Shuman, L.J. & Wolfe, H. (1975) "Mathematical Programming", in Shuman, L.J., Speas, R.D. & Young, J.P. Operations Research in Health Care: A Critical Analysis, Johns Hopkins University Press, 1975.

West, P.A. (1981) "Theoretical & Practical Equity in the National Health Service in England" Social Science & Medicine, Vol.15C, No. 2, June, pp.117-122.

Wolfe, H., (1964) "Multiple Assignment Model for Staffing Nursing Units", PhD thesis, Johns Hopkins University, Baltimore, Md.

ALLOCATION - SUMMARY

Allocation problems relate to typical management decisions where the decision maker has an objective and there are certain constraints which apply that make meeting that objective difficult. The operations research techniques of mathematical, linear and integer programming are available to assist the manager in these circumstances. The simplest of these, linear programming, relates to the situation where the constraints can be expressed in linear form.

General form of Linear Programming Problem:

Objective function: Maximise)
               or Minimise) $c_1x_1 + c_2x_2 + \ldots + c_nx_n$

Subject to Constraints: $a_{11}x_1 + a_{12} + a_{13}x_3 + \ldots + a_{1n}x_n \quad A_1$

$a_{21}x_1 + a_{22}x_2 + \ldots \quad + a_{2n}x_n \quad A_2$

Steps in solving linear programming problems

1. Identify the objective
2. Identify the variables (normally the variables are the things that the decision maker can choose between and will thus be clear from the statement of the objective).
3. Identify the constraints
4. Formulate the problem algebraically i.e. first write down the objective function and then write down the constraint inequations.
5. Solve the problem graphically, by computer or using other means.

REMEMBER: Generally the things that are constraints are not variables, and the things that are variables are not constraints.

An approach to the general solution follows:

Expansion of step 4 from above

(1) First write down the objective function:

OBJECTIVE FUNCTION MAXIMISE: $c_1x_1 + c_2x_2$

(2) Next write down the variable names, and what the constraints relate to in matrix form:

$x_1 \qquad x_2$ First contraint
e.g. staff

$x_1 \qquad x_2$ Second constraint
e.g. money

(3) Then fill in the coefficients as stated in the problem

$a_1x_1 + a_2x_2 \quad A$ (Staff constraint)

$b_1x_1 + b_2x_2 \quad B$ (Money constraint)

(4) Then solve.

6   COMPETITION

Every day we are confronted by problems of varying complexity, some of which require a decision. These problems may occur at work or at home, they may be important or unimportant, the decsions we take may be based on analysis and research or may be based on hunch and guesswork. Administrators facing problems may decide to follow rules or procedures laid down by their superiors or predecessors or they may have to find a completely new solution. Each administrator, however, approaches a problem with his or her own biases and feelings and it is certainly not true to suggest that somehow administrators make 'perfect' decisions unaffected by personal considerations of any kind.

The Nature of a Decision

Every decision has certain common elements. The first of these is obviously the decision maker. Someone (or occasionally, something) has to make a decision. But, by definition, there must be alternatives between which a choice must be made. The alternatives must necessar ily lead to some outcome and very often the decision maker will have preferences concerning these outcomes.

We now have determined the four common elements of all decision problems.

1. The decision maker who chooses between
2. Alternatives which have
3. Outcomes among which he or she has
4. Preferences

Frequently decision making is long, involved and complex. A decision early in a project will affect the choices available later. The decision maker may be able to influence some of the outcomes but others may be based on chance. The decision maker may be able to assign probabilities to the different outcomes or events but then again may not!

Decision Making Techniques

Health service administrators face increasingly diverse problems, which require more complex decision making processes, some of which utilise operations research and computer technology.

Simon (1960) identified two types of decision and decision making techniques: programmed and non programmed. Programmed decisions are of a routine, repetitive nature and hence can be solved by use of routine procedures such as habit, specifying procedures etc. Most organization manuals are designed to cope with this sort of decision. Clearly there are other sorts of decisions which are not routine and are not repetitive: these can be called non-programmed. It is a common mistake of many organizations to forget the existence of non-programmed situations and attempt to specify decisions to be taken in all instances. The administrator is supposed to look askance at 'hunches', 'intuition' etc., yet in many areas of health administration the decisions that will be taken and the actions that will occur are frequently not programmable.

Difficulties arise because it is easy to make a programmed decision, it is easy to instill habits into employees, but how do you train someone for non-programmed decisions which, by their very nature, are one-off events? The principles behind techniques like work study and operations research go some way towards assisting the manager. The problem is, of course, that they cannot possibly be used in every situation and therefore techniques have to be developed to train the manager in making non-programmed decisions and dealing with "one-shot, ill-structured, novel policy decisions".

Applications of operations research and computers can assist in the making of programmed decisions: instead of ordering supplies once a month from habit, operations research models can assist in determining an optimal inventory policy. Several methods have been used to assist managers in acquiring skills in non-programmed decision making. The basis of these is an attempt to understand the human problem solving process rather than an attempt to simulate or copy it.

There are two main techniques for structuring decisions: the first of these is a technique known as the use of "decision trees" or decision theory, the second is the use of game theory.

Decision Trees

Decision trees are useful when outcomes of decisions are affected by chance. They provide a convenient method of portraying the options available and allow a systematic examination of alternatives and thus assist the decision maker to make best use of information available. Many problems are of the type where the decision you make today depends on a whole series of factors that might occur in the future and decisions you might make in the future. It is in these sorts of circumstances that decision theory and decision trees are of most use. The problem is visualised in terms of a tree, with different branches indicating different options and outcomes. A decision tree portrays chance events that may occur as well as future decisions that may be made. Let us now look at a simple example to see how a decision tree works.

Example 6.1

You have invited some people (about 80) over to your place for late afternoon drinks. Your house isn't all that large and you had hoped for a nice day so that your guests could enjoy your very pretty garden. When you wake on the Sunday morning to your great disappointment it is overcast and you are faced with a decision as to where to locate the party.

To keep the problem simple we will limit the choices available to you to inside or outside and the "states of nature" to fine or raining.

The combinations can be seen in a "payoff" table (see Table 6.1).

Table 6.1   Payoff Table for Party

Choices	Events and Outcomes	
	Rain	No rain
Outside	Disaster	Real comfort
Inside	Mild discomfort but happy	Mild discomfort but regrets

This pay-off table is one way of looking at the problem and is quite adequate for a relatively simple problem like the one we have described.

A decision tree also shows the problem. We can use a square to represent a <u>decision point</u> (node) and a circle to represent <u>chance events</u> (nodes).

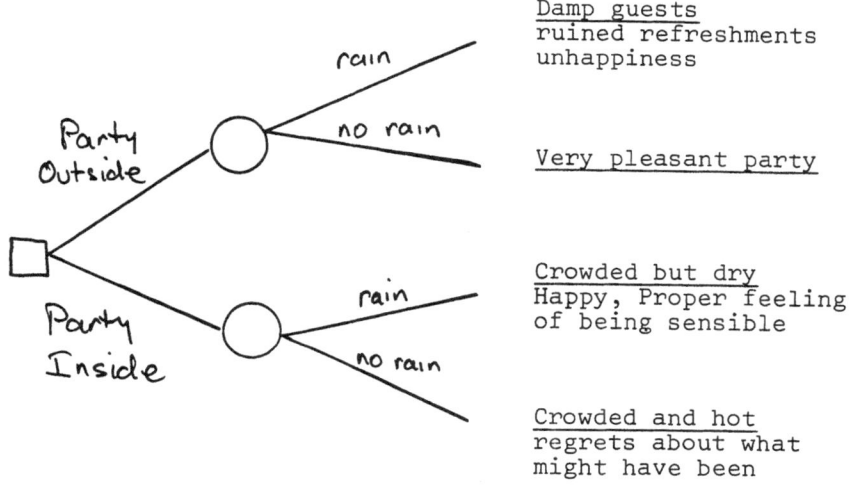

<u>Damp guests</u>
ruined refreshments
unhappiness

<u>Very pleasant party</u>

<u>Crowded but dry</u>
Happy, Proper feeling
of being sensible

<u>Crowded and hot</u>
regrets about what
might have been

<u>Figure 6.1</u>

The party problem described above is the simplest application of the use of decision trees. More complex examples normally involve the introduction of probabilities of the various "states of nature" and valuations being placed on the outcomes. Thus, for example, you might ring up the weather bureau and ascertain that the probability of rain is .3 (and hence, the probability of no rain is .7). Similarly you might decide to rate the various outcomes on a 10 point scale. Clearly the "very pleasant party" is the best outcome and worth 10 points. Similarly the "damp guests" is most unfortunate and worth, say 1 point. The other outcomes have intermediate values. These values can be incorporated in a pay-off table (see Table 6.2).

Table 6.2 Payoff Table with Utilities Shown

Choices	Events and Outcomes Rain	No Rain
Outside	1	10
Inside	6	5

These values can also be incorporated into the decision tree:

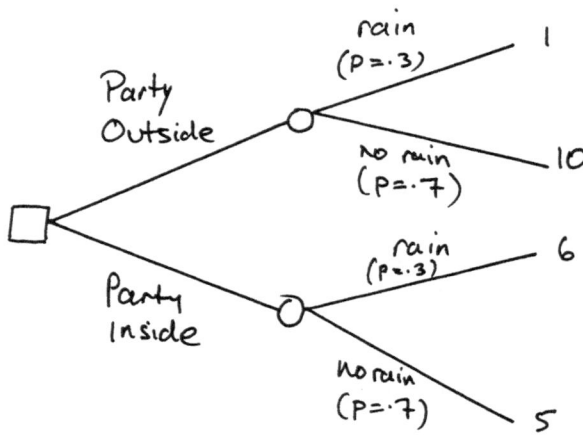

Figure 6.2

Before we evaluate this decision tree it would be useful to refresh your memory about "expected values" . Briefly the expected value of an event which has a number of possible outcomes is simply the sum of the value of each outcome multiplied by the relevant probability. Thus if there are two outcomes, one with probability .3 and value 1, the other with probability .7 and value 10, the expected value of that event is

$$.3 \times 1 + .7 \times 10 = .3 + 7$$
$$= 7.3$$

In general, the Expected Value of an event which has n possible outcomes, each with value x_1 and with probability p_i is $\sum_i x_i p_i$. ('The sum of the probabilities times the outcomes'.)

Returning to our decision tree, the expected value of each of the decisions can be calculated:

$$
\begin{aligned}
E\ (Outside) &= .3 \times 1 + .7 \times 10 \\
&= .3 + 7 \\
&= 7.3
\end{aligned}
$$

$$
\begin{aligned}
E\ (Inside) &= .3 \times 6 + .7 \times 5 \\
&= 1.8 + 3.5 \\
&= 5.3
\end{aligned}
$$

These values can then be incorporated onto the tree (Figure 6.3).

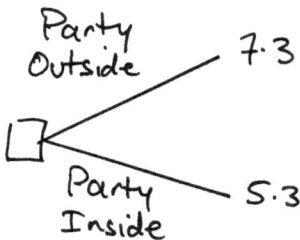

Party
Outside ——— 7.3

Party ——— 5.3
Inside

Figure 6.3

Clearly as the expected value of holding the party outside is
higher than the expected value of holding it inside, one chooses
the former. (You should consider what would happen if the values
of the outcome were somewhat different. For example, if the
outcome of "damp guests" was changed to -10 and all other values
remained unchanged. It should also be stressed that the
assignment of the 'weights' or values represents your own (or the
decision maker's preferences.)

This simplest of decision trees illustrates the general rule for
evaluating decision trees, sometimes known as the "roll back
principle" . Under this system one takes each of the final
outcomes and works backward to:

(i)   average out the values at each chance node (by calculating
       the expected value)

(ii)   at each decision point choose the strategy which will
       maximise the expected future pay-off.

Example 6.2

Kassirer (1976) describes a typical application of decision
analysis in a clinical treatment. In that case a 24 year old
woman had both kidneys removed for bilateral hypernephromas. She
subsequently received a kidney transplant from a cadaver donor
and a splenectomy to correct leukopenia and thrombocytopenia.
Shortly afterwards she was treated with cephalosporin for
Klebsiella sepsis and left lower lobe pneumonia. Kassirer
describes her subsequent condition:

> "On December 3, 1974, she was readmitted to the
> hospital with fever (104.2°F), nausea, vomiting, and
> diarrhea and was found to have rales in the left base
> but no abdominal findings. Over the next several days,
> the symptoms intensified and on December 8 she had
> severe left upper quadrant abdominal pain radiating to
> the left shoulder, generalized abdominal tenderness,
> diminished bowel sounds, splinting of the left chest,
> and poor movement of the left diaphragm. The white
> count was 8900. The diagnosis of subdiaphragmatic
> abscess was considered at this time, and the
> possibility of surgery was first raised...
>
> The choices available to those responsible for the
> patient were either to operate or not to operate, and
> the consequences of both choices can be described
> explicitly. On December 8 there was considerable

uncertainty about the diagnosis of subphrenic abscess. if surgery were carried out (upper branch), a surgically correctable abscess may or may not be present."

Drawing on clinical experience, it was estimated that the probability of a surgically accessible lesion was 0.3.

"Whether the lesion is present or not, the patient may suffer a complication of surgery and the complication may or may not be serious. If a surgically correctable lesion is found, it may or may not be possible to fully evacuate the abscess. If the abscess can be evacuated, the outcome should be excellent: however, if it cannot be fully removed, the lesion may resolve with medical therapy or may lead to sepsis and death."

The outcomes of medical therapy were also evaluated:

"If surgery is not carried out, the patient will presumably recover if a nonsurgical lesion (for example, acute pancreatitis) is the cause of the illness (lowest branch). If surgery is not carried out and the patient actually has a surgically correctable lesion, the outcome would be nearly the same as the lesion described above that was not entirely removed surgically: There would be some chance of spontaneous resolution and some chance of a serious outcome."

These choices can be represented in a decision tree (see Figure 6.4).

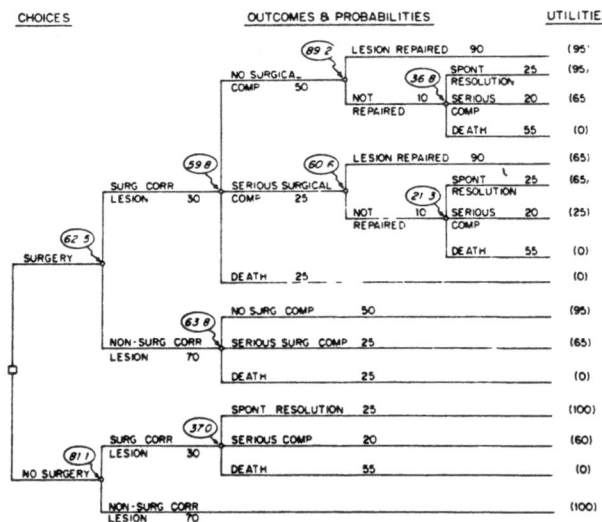

Figure 6.4 Decision tree for a patient suspected of having a subphrenic abscess taken from Kassirer (1976)

The evaluation of the probable outcomes of the two alternatives is undertaken using the standard roll-back technique. Thus for the "no surgery" alternative, the "states of nature" which are present is that either there is a surgically correctable lesion present (probability .3) or there is not (probability .7). If the latter is the case, then the patient will eventually recover anyway with a utility of 100. The expected value of this limb is thus 100 x .7 = 70. On the other hand, if a surgically correctable lesion is present then there are three possible outcomes: there could be spontaneous resolution (probability of .25 and utility of 100); there could be serious complications (probability .2 and utility of 60); or death could eventuate (probability .55 and utility of 0). Calculating the expected value of these outcomes yields an overall expected value of 37.0 (.25 x 100 + .2 x 60 + .55 x 0 = 25 + 12 + 0 = 37.0).

Combining the two states of nature for the no surgery option by calculating the expected value yields an expected value of 81.1 (the probability of the existence of a surgically correctable lesion of .3 multiplied by the expected outcome of that state of nature (37.0) plus the expected value of a non surgically operable lesion (70) = .3 x 37 + 70 = 11.1 + 70 = 81.1).

The calculations involved in the surgery alternative can be performed in a similar manner and yield an expected value of 62.5. Following the rules of the roll-back technique, the alternative with the greater expected value is selected and no surgery would be performed.

Comment on decision analysis

In the discussion so far we have deemphasised two of the crucial problems of decision analysis (or use of decision trees) in the health field: the estimation of probabilities and the assignment of utilities. In most of the clinical applications of decision trees, probabilities have been derived by examining cases of similar problems in the literature or by analysing the experience of patients treated in the clinical unit involved.

Assignment of utilities is essentially a subjective process. Techniques that have been used to assign probabilities in particular instances include combining the judgements of clinicians involved in the case and asking the hospital ethics committee to assign weights. Often the expected values of relevant decision nodes are calculated using several different weights.

Recapitulation

Decisions in administration are often excessively complex and it is difficult to follow through the consequences of a given strategy. The decision maker can portray the options and their effects by use of a decision tree (this is known as decomposition of the problem). The rollback principle is used to evaluate each decision point or chance node. Under this system one takes each outcome and works backward to:

(i) average out the values at each chance node

(ii) at each decision point choose the strategy which will maximise the expected future pay-off.

GAME THEORY

Problems involving the future and unknown outcomes can also be solved by the use of game theory. In this case, instead of displaying information in a decision tree, the information is displayed in tabular form. As with decision trees, game theory portrayal involves acts or strategies, states of nature and outcomes. The outcomes, of course, have certain pay-offs or utilities. The various combination of events are normally portrayed in what has come to be known as a pay-off table (see Table 6.3).

Table 6.3 General Form of Payoff Table

Acts	States of Nature				
	S_1	...	S_j	...	S_n
A_1	r_{11}		r_{1j}		r_{1n}
A_i	r_{11}		r_{ij}		r_{in}
A_m	r_{m1}		r_{mj}		r_{mn}

In this case, the states of nature (S_j) are represented by the various columns and the acts available to the decision maker (A_i) are represented by the rows. The combination of each act and each state of nature is represented by an outcome or pay-off (r_{ij}). In the table, for instance, if you chose act A_1 and state of nature S_1 prevails, then the pay-off or outcome is r_{11}. The outcomes can be expressed in monetary or non-monetary terms. When expressed in non-monetary terms the pay-offs are often called 'utilities'. A simple pay-off table was used in example 6.1.

Risk and Uncertainty

An important distinction made in game theory is between risk and uncertainty. Systems can be divided into four major classes, each category representing an increase in the amount of information known:

1. Non-structured uncertainty   The states of the system are unknown for any given time.

2. Structured uncertainty   The states of the system are known, but we do not know what will be the state of the system for any given time, nor can we ascribe probabilities to the states.

3. Chance or Risk   The states of the system are known as is the probability of each state for any time. If the probabilities do not vary

over time, the system is called 'stationary'; otherwise it is 'non stationary'.

4. Certainty

The states are known and we know the state in which the system will be at any given time.

Thus in some circumstances we may know the outcomes and their associated probabilities for the different states of nature. This sort of problem is said to be one where the decision is taken under <u>risk</u> i.e. for each course of action, the decision maker is aware of the probability distribution of the outcomes. Under conditions of risk there is a set of probabilities $(P_i:P_1, P_2..P_n)$ corresponding to the states of nature $(S_j: S_1, S_2, ..S_n)$. Some situations occur where the decision maker knows precisely what will be the outcome. This situation is known, naturally enough, as <u>certainty</u> and defined as the situation where $P_1 = 1$ and $P_j = 0, \forall j \neq a$ ($\forall$ means 'for all'.)

The case of <u>uncertainty</u> is one where, although the possible states of nature may be known, the probabilities of these are not known. Thus one can neither predict outcomes nor state any information about the likelihood of the various states of nature, other than being able to specify the range of the states of nature which might occur. Many hospital administrators tend to assert that they are forced to make decisions under conditions of uncertainty because they do not believe that it is possible to estimate the probabilities of each of the states of nature. It could be argued, however, that the hospital administrator just is not prepared to seek out the information that would convert a situation of uncertainty to one of risk.

Decision making under certainty is trivial: the future is known! In the next sections we will deal first with decision makig under risk and then, relaxing the assumption that the probability distribution of the states of nature is known, discuss decision making under uncertainty.

Decision Making Under Risk

The simplifying assumption of decisions involving risk is that the probability distribution of the states of nature is known. Nevertheless a number of alternative decision rules have been established which are based on the concept of expected value: the general decision rule is to <u>optimise expected values</u> . By use of expected values, the payoff table will be converted into a single column and the decision is merely one of selecting the optimum value.

Clearly when payoffs can be measured in money terms, the decision is obvious: the values of the outcomes can be reduced to money terms and the maximum expected value selected. It is apparent, however, that in different situations the payoffs could be measured in different ways: evaluation can be in terms of monetary values, opportunity loss or utility.

Monetary Value

In some circumstances the payoffs will be such that they can be accurately evaluated in money terms. A typical problem of this kind is where there are financial returns (or penalties) for each course of action. Using the ordinary statistical rules we can then calculate an expected monetary value (EMV).

It will be recalled in example 6.1, we have two choices available: to hold the party inside or outside. Let us assume we could obtain insurance from the Fairweather Insurance Company to compensate us if it rained. Fairweather have obviously got to place monetary values on the outcomes. They may, for example, draw up the following schedule:

Example 6.3   Fairweather Insurance Company

Premium : $10

Benefits : (i)   If the party is held outside and it rains you will be paid $20.

   (ii)   If the party is held inside and it does not rain you will be paid $12.

   (iii) If the party is held inside and it rains your premium will be refunded.

   (iv)   No payout is made if the party is held outside and it does not rain.

From Fairweather's point of view this can be summarized in the payoff table shown in Table 6.4. (Only the net effect of payout and premium is shown.)

Table 6.4 Fairweather Insurance Payoff Table

Choices	Events	
	Rain	No rain
Outside	-$10	+$10
Inside	0	-$2

Let us now presume that Fairweather check with the weather forecasting service and find that there is a .3 probability of rain on that particular day. Thus, if the client chooses to hold the party outside the expected benefit (to Fairweather Insurance Company) is a net gain of $4 calculated by (probability of rain) x (outcome for rain) + (probability of no rain) x (outcome if no rain) = (.3) x (-$10) + (1 - .3) x ($10) = (-$3) + ($7) = $4. If the client chooses to hold the party inside the expected payout is $1.40 (0 x .3 + -2 x .7 = -1.40). From the insurance company's point of view, they have reduced the competing outcomes to two monetary values and they obviously now hope that the party will be held outside.

Example 6.4 shows a more complicated decision problem.

Example 6.4

Let us assume that we have a payoff table as shown in Table 6.5

Table 6.5   Example Payoff Table

States of Nature

	S_1 $(P = .4)$	S_2 $(P = .5)$	S_3 $(P = .1)$	EMV
A_1	$ 4	$ 8	- $ 2	$ 5.40
A_2	- $ 6	- $ 3	$20	- $ 1.90
A_3	$ 6	- $ 4	$ 6	$ 1.00
A_4	$ 0	$ 0	$ 0	$ 0

Acts is shown to the left of the rows A_2 / A_3.

It is assumed that each of the outcomes can be represented in money terms and an Expected Monetary Value (EMV) calculated.

Thus for Act 1 The Expected Monetary Value is

$4 x .4 + $8 x .5 + (-$2) x .1
= $1.60 + $4.00 + (-$0.20)
= $5.40.

The values for the other acts are calculated in a similar manner. Clearly the expected monetary value is maximised if Act 1 is chosen.

Opportunity Loss

A second way of evaluating outcomes is to consider the opportunity lost. This concept is analogous to that of opportunity cost in economics and represents what you (or the decision maker) missed out on. The opportunity loss is calculated by identifying, for each of the states of nature, the act which would have yielded the optimum payoff. This act has an opportunity loss of 0 for the state of nature. All other acts involve loss of the difference between the (possible) optimum payoff and the payoff that would be received if the other act had been selected. In example 6.4, for instance, if the state of nature was S_1, and you had previously chosen A_3, your return would be $6. A_3 is in fact the best decision you could have made. If, on the other hand you had chosen A_1, your return would have been $4. You would have lost the opportunity of making that additional $2 by making less than the optimal choice. Thus, if the relevant state of nature is S_1, then the opportunity loss for Act A_1 is $2. Similarly, for all other cells, the opportunity loss for an act given a particular state of nature is the difference between the pay off for that combination (of act and state of nature) and the best payoff (over all acts for that state of nature). These opportunity losses can be portrayed in an opportunity loss table (see Table 6.6).

Table 6.6   Example Opportunity Loss Table

States of Nature

	S_1 (P = .4)	S_2 (P = .5)	S_3 (P = .1)	EOL
A_1	$ 2	$ 0	$22	$ 3.00
A_2	$12	$11	$ 0	$10.30
A_3	$ 0	$12	$14	$ 7.40
A_4	$ 6	$ 8	$20	$ 8.40

Clearly in this situation the optimal strategy is to minimise the
expected opportunity loss (EOL).   Thus, in this example, one
would chose Act A_1.   Opportunity loss tables can, of course, be
constructed directly from the formulation of the problem.

Utility

Very often the values of the outcomes of decision problems cannot
be expressed in money terms.   In these situations a numerical
index is developed and different values assigned to the different
outcomes.   Thus, although we may not know the exact valuations of
outcomes in dollars, we have preferences as between outcomes.
The index representing a decision maker's preference is commonly
referred to as the utility index.   (The units are sometimes known
as utils.)

A utility index which only expresses orderings (i.e. act 1 is
better than act 2) is known as an ordinal utility index whereas
one which allows comparison of strengths of preference (i.e. act
1 is 3 times preferable as is act 2) is known as a cardinal
utility index.   Utility measurement can lead to long and involved
discussions but suffice it to say that utility as used in game
theory is normally of a cardinal variety and utilities assigned
by different people need not have the same meanings.

Just as the decision criterion where outcomes are measured in
monetary terms is one of optimising expected monetary value; the
criterion when utilities are used is to optimise expected
utility.   A payoff table showing utilities is derived in the
normal way and expected utility calculated.

Table 6.7   Utility Payoff Table

States of Nature

Acts	A_i	U_{11}	U_{1j}	U_{1n}
	A_i	U_{i1}	U_{ij}	U_{in}
	A_m	U_{m1}	U_{mj}	U_{mn}

The expected utility for Act A_i is $P_1U_{i1} + P_2U_{i2} + \ldots P_nU_{in}$

$$= \sum_{j=1}^{n} P_j U_{ij}$$

(P_j = Probability of occurrence of state of nature j)

The decision criterion can be expressed mathematically as

$$\max \left\{ \sum_{j=1}^{n} P_j U_{ij} \right\}$$

Additional Information

It is useful to compare decisions taken under conditions of risk and those taken under certainty. Clearly if we knew for certain which state of nature were to occur, our choices would be trivial since each act would lead to only one outcome and we would only have to choose the optimal outcome. Such a decision would have a greater expected value than a decision taken under risk.

The Expected Value of Perfect Information (EVPI) is defined as the difference between the expected value of a decision taken under certainty and the expected value of the decision taken under risk. The _expected_ value of a decision taken under certainty is the sum of the probabilities of the various states of nature multiplied by the optimal outcome for the respective states of nature. This is so because the certainty only arises once the state of nature has been determined. Decisions taken under certainty still involve the probabilities of those states of nature occurring.

Now, in example 6.4 if we knew S_1 were to occur, we would obviously choose A_3. Similarly if we knew S_2 were to occur we would choose A_1 and if we knew S_3 were to occur we would choose A_2. What then, is the expected value of a decision taken under certainty? Our payoff is $6 if S_1 occurs since we would choose A_3. The payoffs for the various other strategies available can also be determined. Clearly the _expected_ value of the decision will involve the probabilities that each of these states of nature will occur and hence the expected value under certainty of the decision in 6.4 would be ($6.00 x .4) + ($8.00 x .5) + ($20.00 x .1) = $8.40. Thus if a decision were to be taken under conditions of certainty our expected monetary value would be $8.40. The expected value of the same decision taken under risk has previously been determined as $5.40 The EVPI is thus $8.40 $5.40 = $3.00. It would therefore be worth $3.00 for us to convert a situation of risk to one of certainty and we would be prepared to pay up to $3.00 to discover exactly which state of nature would occur. However, as Horowitz (1965, p.60) puts it:

> "Although it would be nice to have perfect information about the future, there are few soothsayers around to provide it. Quite frequently, however, one can obtain _additional_ information about the likelihood of future outcomes of trials of an event by some sort of sampling or research procedure. This information may not lead us into perfection, but may very well deliver us from evil!"

DECISION MAKING UNDER UNCERTAINTY

Decision making under risk has basically been concerned with decisions taken where the main competitor is nature and the probability distribution of the states of nature are known. We shall now consider 'true' competitive situations in which another individuals' actions affect the outcome of any decision made and thus where the probabilities cannot be predicted or determined. Similar techniques apply where the main competitor is nature but probabilities are unknown. Let us first consider a simple competitive situation into which many of us fall every day.

Example 6.5   The call-back problem

Woop Woop Hospital has an ancient and inefficient switchboard operated by an ancient and inefficient telephonist. As a result, many calls are cut off in the middle of important conversations, one such call was from The Chief Executive Officer of Woop Woop to the Chief Executive Officer of another local hospital. The question now is who should call back first? This problem can be displayed in a pay off matrix as shown in Table 6.8

Table 6.8   Ring-back Problem Payoff Matrix

		CEO – Other	
		Call Back	Wait
CEO	Call back	0	1
	Wait	1	0

The utilities have been assigned such that a reconnection of the call is equally desirable to both and a wait leaves both unaffected. Since this case is a completely symmetrical problem, game theory offers no clue to the solution and other decision rules (such as who initiated the call) are followed. It can, however, be useful in other situations.

ANALYSIS OF GAMES OR DECISIONS UNDER UNCERTAINTY

A number of writers have analysed games to attempt to ascertain how decisions are made, what are the optimal outcomes etc. We shall look at their conclusions in two areas. First, some writers have attempted to analyse the strategies that a decision maker may adopt. For example, a pessimistic decision maker can be expected to act differently from an optimistic decision maker. Various decision criteria have been developed which reflect different personality traits and different methods of decision making.

Secondly, some writers have analysed solutions of games; for instance whether a particular game has a stable solution (i.e. there is no incentive for a decision maker to change the action (or strategy) decided upon, and whether particular actions or strategies are bound to be chosen and what to do if there is no best solution.

Decision criteria

Several criteria have been developed to assist managers in deciding problems of uncertainty. The methods can apply to both games and decisions taken against nature. Let us consider an example (based on one formulated by Mitchell (1972)).

Example 6.6   Health Planning

A health planning agency has the opportunity of deciding on the location of a new hospital. There are, as yet, no figures for demand or need but the agency has narrowed the choice down to two towns, A or B. If it is decided to locate the hospital in either town there are three possible outcomes:

(i)   The bulk of the admissions will come from the town in which the hospital is sited.

(ii)   50% of the admissions will come from each town.

(iii)   The bulk of the admission will come from the other town.

The alternative decisions can be described as a_1 and a_2, the possible states of nature as S_1, S_2 and S_3. A payoff matrix (Table 6.9) can be calculated, taking into account the preferences of agency staff and other extraneous variables.

Table 6.9   Bed Planning Payoff Matrix

	S_1 bulk of admissions from Town A	S_2 admissions evenly divided	S_3 bulk of admiss- ions from Town B
A_1 (locate hospital in Town A)	100 (very good)	40	0 (very bad)
A_2 (locate hospital in Town B)	10 (bad)	60	80 (good)

This payoff matrix shows the utility of each of the outcomes (remember, that these are the health planning agency's estimations and may not be those of the inhabitants of town B). We can also calculate a 'regret' matrix (Table 6.10). The regret incurred in a decision is the amount by which the decision made falls short of the best possible decision (i.e. the opportunity loss). For example, if the bulk of the admissions were to come from Town B, and the hospital had been located in town A, the regret would be 80 (the best possible) -0 or 80. If, on the other hand the hospital had been located in town B the regret would be zero since that would be the best possible outcome.

Table 6.10   Regret Matrix for Bed Planning Problem

	S_1	S_2	S_3
A_1	0 (very good)	20	80 (bad)
A_2	90 (very bad)	0 (very good)	0 (very good)

As indicated above, decision theorists have identified several different criteria for making decisions. Using the values given above, let us now look at these different criteria that can be employed to make a decision.

Bernoulli, Laplace or Insufficient Reason

The simplest way of dealing with uncertainty is to assume that it does not exist! This is done by converting the problem under review to one of risk by assigning probabilities to the various outcomes. As Laplace (a famous mathematician) said, 'If I know nothing of nature but the states it can take, I assume these states to be equiprobable'. Thus the 'principle of insufficient reason' assumes that all possible values of the state of nature are equally likely and advises us to select the one which has the highest average utility.

That is, if for a mutually exclusive and jointly exhaustive listing of states of nature, there is no evidence to suggest that one state is more likely than another, we then assume that all are equally probable and assign the same probability of occurrence to each. The difficulty with this criterion is, of course, the listing of the mutually exclusive and exhaustive states of nature.

In example 6.6, the health planning agency could assume that each of the three outcomes concerning admission patterns are equally likely and calculate the utility as if we were considering a decision taken under risk. The calculation would yield a utility for A_1 (locating the hospital in town A) of 1/3 (100+40+0) = 46.66 and for A_2 of 1/3 (10+60+80) = 50. The health planning agency would then choose to locate the hospital in town B.

Maximin or the Wald criterion

Occasionally a manager or decision maker can be regarded as a pessimist and will assume that, whatever he or she does, it will be wrong. The decision maker assumes, for example, that whatever strategy is followed the worst possible outcome will occur. The decision maker's strategy would then be to try and 'get the best of a bad bunch', and he or she would try and get the maximum of all the minimum! This criterion is often named after another famous mathematician, Abraham Wald.

Thus in example 6.6, if the health planning agency followed strategy A_1 and located the hospital in Town A, being pessimist, the agency would assume that the bulk of the admission would come from Town B and the utility would be 0. If on the other hand, the agency had decided to locate the hospital Town B, the worst thing that could happen would be for the bulk of the admissions to come from Town A in which case the utility is 10. Since the agency expects (pessimistically) the worst outcome of either strategy, the best course of action is to locate the hospital in town B for a utility of 10.

Minimax Regret or the Savage Criterion

Of course the true blue pessimist is a rare character but another type is Mr. (or Ms.) 'Might-have-been'. Some people often look at alternatives and consider the possible opportunities. A decision criterion that can be used if this is thought applicable is minimax regret . The decision maker would consider the maximum 'regret' that each of the strategies would cause and then act to minimise this amount. Thus in Example 6.6, if the health planning agency had decided to locate the hospital in A, the regret matrix (Table 6.10) shows us that the maximum regret would occur if the bulk of the admissions came from town B. Agency staff would then dream wistfully of having located the hospital in town B. If, however, the agency had located the hospital in B the maximum regret would occur if the bulk of the admissions came from A. The agency could minimise maximum regret by choosing to locate the hospital in A. The decision is different from that taken under a maximum strategy. This criterion is often attributed to a mathematician named Savage.

Maximax

Returning to the utility matrix, a decision criterion that could be adopted is to maximise the best possible alternative i.e. maximise the maximum utility. In example 6.6, we would see that the best possible outcome is to locate the hospital in A and have the bulk of the admissions coming from town A. Chou (1972) draws attention to the fact that it is useful if you are sufficiently well off (or insured) that you do not have to consider the worst alternative.

> 'The maximax rule, well suited to a confirmed optimist who always looks through rose-coloured glasses, considers only the most glittering possible reward and ignores all other contingencies. This rule is quite appropriate where the decision maker can well sustain the worst penalties. The maximax rule, like the maximin, ignores all intermediate pay-offs, even though some may be only negligibly lower'.

Hurcwicz or Coefficient of Optimism

Some decision makers prefer neither the high road nor the low road and prefer to take a middle course. One method of giving some weight to the best outcomes and some weight to the worst outcome is the hurcwicz criterion . A coefficient of optimism, c, is determined ranging from 0 (for a complete pessimist) to 1 (for a complete optimist). (For a discussion of how to calculate the hurcwicz coefficient see either Peston & Coddington (1968) or Mitchell (1972)). Using the hurcwicz criterion we then calculate a weighted average of the outcomes for each act. Thus for act A_1 for example, we calculate $H(A_1)$ by multiplying the best possible outcome from that act by the coefficient of optimism and adding that to the product of the worst possible outcome and (1-coefficient). The formula for calculating the hurcwicz index is thus $(H(A_1) = c$ max $Uij + (1-C)$ min Uij. The decision criterion is to maximise $H(A_i)$. It can easily be seen that in the case of the perfect optimist (c=1), the hurcwicz criterion is identical to maximax. On the other hand, in the case of the perfect pessimist, hurcwicz is identical to maximin. Instead of first determining a coefficient of optimism and then evaluating the hurcwicz indices, an alternative approach which can be followed when using the hurcwicz criterion is to treat c, the coefficient of optimism, as a variable and use simultaneous equations to find the values of c for which each alternative is preferred. In example 6.6, the health planning agency might place itself on an optimism-pessimism scale:

0	1/3	1/2	2/3	1
Pessimist				Optimist

The agency, for example, could assume it has a coefficient of 2/3. We can calculate $H(A_1)$ & $H(A_2)$ for the hospital location problem as follows:

$$H(A_1) = .66 \times 100 + (1-.66) \times 0 = 66.66$$
$$H(A_2) = .66 \times 80 + (1-.66) \times 10 = 56.66$$

The health planning agency would therefore choose the maximum of the two, and locate the hospital in A.

The alternative, simultaneous equations approach, can also be undertaken. In this case:

$$H(A_1) = c \times 100 + (1-c) \times 0$$
$$= 100C$$
$$H(A_2) = c \times 80 + (1-c) \times 10$$
$$= 80c - 10c \times 10$$
$$= 70c + 10$$

now $H(A_1) > H(A_2)$

if $100c > 70c + 10$
i.e. if $30c > 10$
$c > 0.333$

Act 2 would be preferred to Act 1 if our coefficient of optimism is less than 0.333. Act 1 would be preferred to Act 2 if our coefficient of optimism is greater than 0.333. We would be indifferent between the choices (i.e. the hurcwicz indices would be identical) if our coefficient of optimum is equal to 0.233. (When using this approach it is important to remember that $0 < c < 1$).

Recapitulation

The various criteria can be expressed mathematically by regarding the utility of the ith act (row) in the face of the jth state of nature (column) as U_{ij} and recalling that the maximum of a series (r_i) can be indicated $\max (r_i)$. The decision criteria can then be stated:

Bernoulli
$$\max_i \frac{1}{n} \sum_j U_{ij}$$

Maximin
$$\max_i \min_i (U_{ij})$$

Minimax Regret
Regret: $R_{ij} = \max_r (U_{rj} - U_{ij})$

Decision is to select
$$\min_i \max_j (R_{ij})$$

Maximax
$$\max_i \max_j (U_{ij})$$

Hurcwicz

$$\max_i H(A_i) = c \max_j U_{ij} + (1-c) \min_j U_{ij}$$

Solution of Games

Before we move to a consideration of some of the uses of competition three further notions, concerned with the 'solution' of games, will be considered: saddle points, dominance and mixed strategies.

Saddle Points

In some games where one decision maker is playing against another decision maker (other than nature), the situation may arise where there is no incentive for either player to change strategies. The game is thus at an equilibrium point and the value of the payoff at that point is known as the value of the game . If both players adopt a maximin strategy this can occur when a given payoff is simultaneously a minimum of a row and the maximum of a column. This point is normally known as the saddle point of the payoff matrix because of its appearance when plotted in three dimensions.

It can be shown that if there is more than one saddle-point in any two-person game, the payoffs must be equal. In summary, then, a saddle point exists if and only if the maximum of the row minima equals the minimum of the column maxima. If it does exist, the game is said to be strictly determined since both players will obtain an acceptable solution.

Dominance

A dominating strategy is a strategy which is always preferred by a player, i.e. it is a strategy which is 'better' than any other available. An Act a_1 is thus said to be 'dominant' over another act a_r if, for each possible state of nature, a_k leads to a payoff which is at least as high as that for a_R and for at least 1 state of nature a_k leads to a higher payoff than a_r. When examining payoff matrices where a dominating strategy exists, all dominated strategies can be ignored (and there is thus no need to calculate expected values, row maxima etc. for those strategies).

Mixed Strategies

Saddle points and games involving dominance do not normally have any probabilistic elements. A decision maker can, however, select strategies at random (but according to a specific probability distribution) such that the decision maker is indifferent to the outcome. By so doing, this would ensure that the expected minimum gain (statistically determined) is in excess of the minimum gain obtained using maximin. This sort of procedure is known as a mixed strategy. Thus, if a decision criterion yields identical (optimal) values for several acts, the decision maker would follow a mixed or random strategy covering the acts.

APPLICATIONS TO HEALTH ADMINISTRATION

Decision theory and game theory can be applied to health administration and medical care in much the same manner as to business and government administration. One major area of application of decision analysis and decision trees is in clinical decision making. A number of writers have been struck by the similarities between making a diagnosis using information supplied by tests, symptoms and examinations and the Bayesian process and decision trees. Barnoon and Wolfe (1972) and Krischer (1980) have reviewed a number of applications of statistics to the diagnostic process and the use of Bayesian analysis to evaluate clinical decision making. Fries (1981) also includes a section concerning applications of operations research in medical management - most of the studies to which he refers are based on decision analysis.

Clinicians are often faced with questions such as the one considered by Ginsberg and Offensend (1968) in their study of back pain:

> 'Should the physicians attempt some more diagnostic tests (and if so, which ones); wait for new symptoms to appear; or should they start treating the patient for one of the diseases he might possibly have?'

In this particular case, the time element was crucial and there were difficulties associated with additional tests. Ginsberg and Offensend reported that the problem was analysed using a decision tree to highlight the alternatives and associated outcomes.

An important review of surgical practice in the United States (Bunker et al, 1977) included a number of papers which used decision theory to evaluate decision making in surgery. The papers included consideration of appendectomy (Pliskin and Taylor, and Neutra); hypertensive disease (McNeil); inguinal herniorrhaphy (Neuhauser) and coronary artery bypass surgery (Weinstein et al). Warner & Holloway (1978) also includes a number of examples of the use of decision trees. Clarification of the medical decision making process using decision theory can facilitate use of computers to model or assist the diagnostic or treatment process. Rogers, Ryack and Moeller (1979) provides a comprehensive literature review of this area.

Bayesian analysis was also used by Flagle and Lechat (1963) to analyse the utility of a screening programme for leprosy. In this case there was a screening test, which predicted the true state of nature which a particular probability and several strategies for further investigation of the population (hospitalisation, outpatient treatment or no treatment).

A similar analysis was used by Walton (1964) in evaluating a 'steering clinic'. Such a clinic is used to 'steer' self referred patients to the appropriate outpatient clinic. Walton developed a questionnaire which, analysed using a Bayesian framework, can quickly facilitate diagnosis. A further screening example is that of Nunez (1969) who compared continuous screening programes to 'one-off' programs and no program at all. Nunez developed loss tables and prepared a decision tree indicating the outcomes and probabilities of each of the strategies.

A non-medical study, but one which still has relevance for the
health administrator is that of Hartmann and Moglewer (1967)
which provided a mathematical model, based on game thoretic
principles, for the selection of research proposals. As the
difference between deciding upon R & D proposals in business and
their counterparts in the health field is negligible, the
procedures used could well be applied by health research funding
organisations.

Duckett (1977) analysed the use of game theory to assist the
rostering of nurses on public holidays. The nurse administrator
must roster, say, between 1 and 4 nurses with no knowledge of the
likely demand for care. Such a situation is a classic
competition problem of decision making under uncertainty.

Probably the most interesting application of game theory is in
planning and forecasting. Despite the implicit assumptions of
many health services planners it is difficult to forecast the
future - and this fact applies to population projections as well
as roulette wheels and horse racing. Two examples will suffice.
Pollard (1975) analysed projections of live births in the United
Kingdom made in 1955, 1960, 1965 & 1970. The projections for
1995 ranged from about 700,000 births (1955 projection) to
1,500,000 births (1965 projection).

The projections resulted in widely differing estimates of greatly
differing accuracy. If the planning of health facilities or the
supply of health personnel had been based on the 1955 estimates,
there would have been a significant underprovision.

An Australian example is in the Borrie report (Australia, 1975)
which caused a drastic revision of estimates of the size of the
future population. But the Borrie report was based on certain
assumptions about, for example, fertility rates and net
immigration. Even ignoring the criticisms that have been made
of these assumptions by, for example, Hall (1976), different
assumptions about fertility and immigration rates lead to
population sizes in 2085 of between 18 million and 75 million.
The exact estimate of future population that is used in planning
depends both on the planners assumptions about fertility rates
and the Government's decisions about immigration rates.

Peston and Coddington (1968) formulated a game theory application
with two states of nature (growth rate of population of a% and
b%) and two acts: a high or low rate of provision of hospital
beds. Given the difficulties in making accurate population
projections, this example thus has clear applicability. The
future population of most countries is not known with certainty
and, in most cases, different population sizes can be regarded as
different states of nature. The same problems apply to planning
for small areas, as the projections of population for sub-state
areas suffer from even greater variability than do the population
projections for a country as a whole. The planner, when choosing
the population he or she will plan for is clearly ascribing
probabilities to the various outcomes on the basis of his or her
own beliefs or values! This is not necessarily undesirable but
these beliefs and values should be made explicit. Harrington
(1977) includes a discussion of the use of decision theory in
forecasting. Grimes (1974) discusses an application of game

theory in regional hospital planning.

Game theory can also be used to explain the behaviour of individuals and groups in an organisation. Although most of the applications of it have been confined to competitive market situations, the basic principles can be easily applied to non-profit competition amongst health care institutions. Mattson (1969) has described a decision theory approach used in the selection of medical students.

He considers a situation where a medical school has more applications than positions available. Clearly each applicant is either accepted or rejected and if accepted, graduates in minimum time; graduates later or does not graduate at all! Mattson then specified probabilities for graduation for each of six groups of students, (the groups are selected on residential and academic grounds). Costs for each of the groups are estimated and an expected value for each group determined. Mattson then develops the model in the traditional manner and concludes as follows:

> 'The author feels the article represents a gauntlet thrown down before all individuals having a part in medical student selection procedures. In essence, it says that any rational policy of selecting medical students must be based on the concepts and the model presented. The challenge is not so much to adopt the model, since the author feels that the model is already used on an informal basis. Rather the challenge is to make explicit the definitions of categories, treatment costs, outcome values, and other decisional elements in order that there may be subject to examination and that existing selection strategies may be reviewed in the context of these definitions'.

The same strongly worded statement could be made about a number of aspects of operations research and their application. Decision theory and game theory are, as yet, rarely applied to hospitals and health care generally but is this because they are not relevant or that hopital managers are not ready for them? Do hospital managers feel so unsure of their positions that they must obfuscate rather than elucidate?

The words of Cronbach and Gleser (1957) may help to answer this:

> 'The assignment of values to outcomes is the Achilles heel of decision theory. Once outcomes have been evaluated, one can proceed in a fully rigorous fashion to compare particular decisions of general strategies. The evaluation of outcomes, however, seems often to be arbitrary and subjective, leading one to question whether any of the conclusions from decision theory can be trustworthy if the starting point itself is open to dispute.
>
> The most telling answer to this objection is to point out that decision theory invokes no more subjective evaluation than does any method of arriving at courses of action. Every choice between actions involves evaluation, and every doctrine or set of principles embodies value judgement. ...The unique feature of

decision theory or utility theory is that it specifies evaluations by means of a payoff matrix or by conversion of the criterion to utility units. The values are thus plainly revealed and open to criticism. This is an asset rather than a defect of this system, as compared with systems where value judgements are imbedded and often pass unrecognized.'

REFERENCES

Ackoff, R.L. & Sasieni, M.W., (1968) Fundamentals of Operations Research, Wiley, 1968.

Australian National Population Inquiry (Chairman: W.D. Borrie) (1975) Population & Australia: A Demographic Analysis & Project, Vol. 1, AGPS.

Barnoon, S. & Wolfe, H., (1972) Measuring the Effectiveness of Medical Decions, Charles C. Thomas, III.

Bunker, J.P., Barnes, B.A. & Mosteller, F. (eds.) (1977) Costs, Risks and Benefits of Surgery, Oxford UP.

Chou, Y., (1972) Probability & Statistics for Decision Making, Holt, Rinehart & Winston.

Cronbach, L.J. & Gleser, G.C., (1957) Psychological Tests & Personnel Decisions, Uni. of Ill. Press.

Duckett, S.J., (1977) 'Nurse Rostering with Game theory', Journal of Nursing Administration, VII(1): 58-59, January.

Flagle, C.D. & Lechat, M.F., (1973) 'Statistical Decision Theory & The Selection of Therapeutic Strategies in Public Health', Proceedings of 3rd Inst. Conf. in OR. pp.194-203.

Fries, B.E., (1981) Applications of Operations Research to Health Care Delivery Systems: A Complete Review of the Periodical Literature (Lecture Notes in Medical Informatics No. 10), Springer Verlag.

Ginsberg, C.D. & Offensend, F., (1968) 'An Application of Decision Theory to a Medical Diagnosis - Treatment Problem', Rand P-3786, also published as Ginsberg, C.D. & Offensend, F.L. 'An Application of Decision Theory to a Medical Diagnosis Treatment Problem', IEEE Transactions on Systems Science & Cybernetics , Vol. SSC4, No. 3, pp.355-362, September.

Grimes, R.M., Allen, C.L., Sparling, T.R. & Weiss, G., (1974) 'Use of Decision Theory in Regional Planning, Health Services Research , Vol. 9, No. 1, pp.73-78, Spring.

Hall, A.R., 'Of Baby Booms & Marriage Slumps', (1976) Economic Record , 52(1):36-51, March.

Harrington, M.B., (1977) 'Forecasting Areawide Demand for Health Care Services: A Critical Review of Major Techniques & Their Application', Inquiry , XIV(3):254-268, September.

Hartman, F. & Moglewer, S., (1967) 'Allocation of Resources to Research Proposals', Management Science (Theory) , 14:85-110.

Kassirer, J.P. (1976) 'The Principles of Clinical Decision Making: An Introduction to Decision Analysis' Yale Journal of Biology & Medicine , Vol. 49, pp.149-164.

Krischer, J.P. (1980) 'An Annotated Bibliography of Decision Analytic Applications to Health Care' Operations Research Vol.

28, No. 1, pp.97-113, Jan-Feb.

Mattson, D.E., (1969) 'Use of a Formal Decision Theory Model in Selection of Medical Students', Journal of Medical Education , 44:964-73, October.

McNeil, B.J., (1977) 'The value of diagnostic aids in patients with potential surgical problems' in Bunker, J.P. et al (eds.), pp.77-90.

Mitchell, G.H. (ed.), (1972) Operations Research: Techniques & Examples , English Uni. Press.

Neuhauser, D. (1977) 'Elective inguinal herniorrhaphy versus truss in the elderly' in Bunker, J.P. et al (eds.), pp.223-239.

Neutra, R. (1977) 'Indications for the surgical treatment of suspected acute appendicitis: a cost effectiveness approach' in Bunker, J.P. et al (eds.), pp.277-309.

Nunez, A.F., (1969) 'Disease Detection Under Uncertainty: An Applied Model', in Weber, C.E. & Peters, G., Management Action: Models of Admin. Decisions , International Textbook Co.

Peston, M. & Coddington, A., (1968) 'The Elementary Ideas of Game Theory', CAS Occasional Paper No. 7 .

Pliskin, N. & Taylor, A.K. (1977) 'General principles: cost benefit and decision analysis' in Bunker, J.P. et al (eds.), pp.5-27.

Pollard, J.H., (1975) 'Modelling Human Populations for Projection Purposes: Some of the Problems & Challenges, Australian Journal of Statistics , 17(2):63-76, June.

Rogers, W., Ryack, B. & Moeller, G. (1979) 'Computer-aided Medical Diagnosis: Literature Review' International Journal of Biomedical Computing 10: 4 (August) pp.267-289.

Simon, H.A., (1960) The New Science of Management Decision , Harper. 1960.

Thomas, H.A., (1972) Decision Theory and the Manager , Pitman.

Walton, W.E., (1964) 'Modern Decision Theory Applied to Medical Diagnosis', Ph.D. Thesis, Johns Hopkins University.

Warner, D.M. & Holloway, D.C., (1978) Decision Making and Control for Health Adminitration: The Management of Qualitative Analysis , Health Administration Press.

Weinstein, M.C., Pliskin, J.S. & Stason, W.B., (1977) 'Coronary artery bypass sugery: decision and policy analysis' in Bunker, J.P. et al (eds.), pp.342-371.

COMPETITION - A SUMMARY

A decision has four basic elements: there is

1. The decision maker who chooses between

2. Alternatives which have

3. Outcomes among which he or she has

4. Preferences

The "competition" techniques dealt with include

(a) decision trees

(b) game theory.

The types of problems include situations of risk (where the outcomes and probability of the outcomes are known) and situations of uncertainty where although the outcomes are known the probability distributions are not.

(a) Decision trees are most useful when the outcome of a decision is affected by chance and there are sequential decisions involved (e.g. if I decide A, three different outcomes can occur, I have then to make another decision etc.). The method used in solving/evaluating decision trees is the roll-back technique by which we:

(i) calculate the expected value of each chance node, and

(ii) choose the optimum strategy at each decision point.

(b) Game theory uses pay-off tables to help us come to our decision. When we have a decision under risk solutions can be calculated on the basis of expected values. In situations of uncertainty we can use certain decision criteria (maximin, minimax regret, maximax, hurcwicz, bernoulli) bit we should also look for saddle points, dominating strategies and mixed strategies.

(i) Bernoulli, Laplace or Insufficient Reason

Assume that each state of nature is equally likely, then calculate the expected value and then choose the act which yields the maximum expected value. Algebraically, if the utility of the ith act (row) in the face of the jth state of nature (column) is U_{ij} we choose $\max_{i} \frac{1}{n} \underset{j}{\leqq} U_{ij}$ (n rows maximum of expected value

(ii) Maximin or Wald criterion

This is the pessimist approach. For each act calculate the worst outcome and then choose the act which leads to the best of their worst outcomes (i.e. choose the maximin of the row minima).

Algebraically we choose: $\max_i \min_j (U_{ij})$

(iii) Minimax Regret

This is the decision criterion for Mr. Might-have-been. We first calculate the regret matrix [for each column we identify the best act; in the regret matrix this act has a value zero. For each other act we calculate the difference between the maximum value (i.e. the value of the best act) and the act under consideration; this difference is then the value for that act (for that column) in the regret matrix.

Algebraically Regret: $R_{ij} = \max_r (U_{rj} - U_{ij})$]

Having calculated the regret matrix, we identify, for each act, what is the most we would ever miss out on (i.e. the row maximum). We then choose the act which will lead us to minimise this value. i.e. we choose the <u>mini</u>mum of the row <u>maxi</u>ma (of the) <u>Regret</u> matrix.

Algebraically we choose: $\min_i \max_j (R_{ij})$

(iv) Maximax

This is the decision criterion for the optimist. We identify the best possible outcome of each act and then choose the act which leads to the best of those bests i.e. we choose to <u>maxi</u>mise the row <u>maxi</u>ma.

Algebraically we choose to: $\max_i \max_j (U_{ij})$

(v) Hurcwicz or Coefficient of Optimism

This is the decision criterion for the middle road. There are two ways to calculate this, although each involves the calculation of the hurcwicz index. The first is to choose what we regard as our coefficient of optimism (e.g. .4) and calculate the index using that value. The index is calculated by identifying for each act the maximum value and multiplying that value by the coefficient and then identifying the minimum value and multiplying that by 1 minus the coefficient. The index is the sum of those values. If the coefficient is .4, then for each act the hurcwicz index is .4x (max value) + .6x (min value).

Algebraically $H(a_i) = c \max_j U_{ij} + (1 - c) \min_j (U_{ij})$
where c is the coefficient of optimism.

Having calculated the hurcwicz coefficient for each act, you choose the act which has the maximum coefficient.

Algebraically you choose $\max\limits_{j} H(A_i)$

The second method is to treat the hurcwicz coefficient as a variable and calculate the algebraic value of each act in terms of c. One can then calculate the values of c for which each of the acts might be chosen e.g. you might discover the act 1 is chosen if $c \not> .3$; act 2 if c is between .1 & .3; act 3 if c is less than .1 and act 4 would never be chosen.

7   SEARCH

An important class of operations research problems is concerned
with identifying deviations from previously determined standards
or isolating changes in quality. These problems are not so much
concerned with what decision to make but rather with determining
what or how much information should be collected, and how the
information should be analysed and presented.

Although search problems are most commonly applied to quality
control situations, the same principles can be applied to many
other areas of health administration and planning. Search
problems were first encountered in quality control situations in
factories and laboratories but exactly the same principles can be
applied in the clinical management review procedures utilized to
evaluate the quality of medical care.

The need to control the quality of any process (such as
laboratory tests) arises in all cases where variations may from
time to time give rise to output which is of unsatisfactory
quality. A quality control system should provide for the
measurement of relevant quality related factors or attributes
and should enable the observed values to be compared with
pre-determined standards. Information about the comparisons
should be fedback to management to enable remedial action to be
taken where necessary.

Two aspects of an efficient quality control system need to be
emphasized. First, inspection of all items in most circumstances
would be extremely costly, and so it is usual to employ a
sampling procedure which does not necessitate 100% inspection.
Secondly, it is highly desirable that only the exceptions to the
normal behaviour of the system should be reported to management.
Otherwise management may be swamped with data which mainly report
acceptable results. This is an illustration of the general
principle of management by exception.

A decision management has to make is to balance the cost of
sampling (the greater the size of the sample, the more costly it
is yet the more reliable it is) and the cost of missing out on
important deviations. Statistical quality control techniques
provide a basis for achieving both these objectives. Briefly
statistical techniques are used to determine appropriate methods
of sampling and these are then portrayed on a chart. The data
are obtained from a sample of observations and the charts permit
attention being focussed on those results which appear to lie
outside the ordinary range of variation in quality.

There are, of course, many ways of classifying search problems. Ackoff and Sasieni (1968) suggest two major groupings:

1. Qualitative or quantitative
2. Distributive or collective

The two groupings refer to different stages of the search procedure.

If we observe an element of a population or an element chosen from a process we can look at that element in qualitative or quantitative terms. In qualitative terms we may have to decide whether an item is acceptable or not acceptable, whether it is good or bad. In quantitative terms, we could measure the element along a continuum - what is its diameter, its weight, its hardness.

Having looked at the element we may then make a decision concerning the whole batch from which is was drawn. This is known as a collective decision. On the other hand, we may look at the single element and apply our decision to that element alone and draw no conclusions about the remainder of the population. If this approach is taken our approach is said to be distributive.

Search procedures are a practical way of implementing management by exception. Clearly variations in the quality (or amount) of the output may occur for a number of reasons - some are due to chance variations and some are assignable. Wild (1972) points out:-

> "Chance causes rarely result in large variations, and since they occur for many reasons and in a random manner their occurrence can be described by a statistical probability distribution. Assignable causes, such as differences or changes in materials or machines, or differences between operators, usually account for larger variations, and since such causes can be identified, their occurrence and effects can be controlled."

Search problems rely on control charts to identify those variations in a process which are unlikely to be due solely to chance: assignable variation can, therefore, be highlighted and examined.

As indicated above, the optimum sampling procedure adopted should take into account costs associated with inspection of items, with investigating possible out of control situations and with failing to detect the process being out of control. Less frequent sampling, smaller samples and wider limits will tend to increase the total costs associated with failing to detect out of control situations, but will reduce total inspection costs and the costs of investigating possible out of control situations. In principle the criterion to be used in setting up an efficient quality control procedure is that the expected value of the three types of costs involved should be minimized by selecting the appropriate combination of frequency of sampling, sample size, and width of control limit. In practice, the costs involved are extremely difficult to estimate, especially those associated with investigating out of control situations, and with failing to remedy out of control situations. The latter may be measured by the amount of spoilage which results from failing to detect a change in the system, but the actual cost which arises will depend on the stage at which the defect is actually detected.

The expected value of the cost therefore depends on the probabilities of the defect being detected at all subsequent stages of production, distribution, etc. For this reason there is little point in this case in developing an explicit cost function. However, the cost considerations mentioned above provide a guide for trial and error experimentation when a control system has been developed. Thus if inspection costs are unduly high, the frequency of sampling may be reduced and then a further check should be made on whether the costs associated with defective items remaining undetected have risen to a disproportionate level. A full consideration of the operations research technique of search theory involves estimation of these cost functions. These procedures will not be discussed here, as we shall concentrate on the techniques associated with sampling.

QUALITY CONTROL

The basic theory of quality control is derived directly from the theory of sampling and of the sampling distribution of means. If we first recall that for a population that is normally distributed (with mean μ and standard deviation σ), 68.26% of the values fall within the range $\mu \pm \sigma$, 95.45% of the values fall within the range $\mu \pm 2\sigma$, and 99.73% of the values fall within the range $\mu \pm 3\sigma$, it can quickly be seen that only a very small percentage of values lie outside the range $\mu \pm 3\sigma$: by concentrating our attention on the values that do lie outside this range, we are almost certainly not going to be looking for events or values caused by chance variations. The choice of whether to use limits based on two standard deviations or three standard deviations from the mean is normally taken in the early stages of developing a control system. It partly reflects implicit valuations of the cost of failure to detect out of control situations (or, conversely, importance of insuring that deviation from the mean is not too great).

The basic principles of quality control are implemented by control charts. We plot the values of various elements on the chart to discover whether the values fall into an acceptable range. The "elements" plotted may vary, most commonly they could be:

(i)   single values of an element sampled
(ii)   values of the mean of a small sample
(iii) values of a certain attribute (e.g. percentage defective)
(iv)   number of defects found.

Both quantitative and qualitative examples can be handled using statistical control charts. The decision, of course, may be either distributive or collective. It should be especially noted that when a small sample is taken the mean is only one indicator of performance: it is common to plot the range of the sample or

the standard deviation in addition to the mean. Methods of
plotting variations in the range are somewhat similar to those
used for plotting the mean but will not be discussed here. We
shall, however, consider the four types of plotting listed
above.

(i) <u>Single Values</u>

Sometimes we can be sure that the population from which we are
sampling is normally distributed. Thus, if we plot the values of
single samples from that population, they will be distributed as
a normal curve, with the same mean and standard deviation as the
parent population.

In these cases, the quality control chart is based on taking
samples of the output of the process at regular intervals and
plotting the values on a graph. In this case the samples are of
size 1. If the process is "under control" the variations of the
sample around the population mean (referred to as the <u>process
average</u>) will be due to chance (random) causes, and less than 5
per 100 will lie outside the $\mu \pm 2\sigma$ bounds and less than 3 per
1000 outside the $\mu \pm 3\sigma$ bounds.

Occasionally, however, a change in the system will give rise to a
significant change in the pattern of output, leading to either
too great or to persistent a shift in the values of the samples.
The "change in the system" may be a reflection of a mechanical
malfunction, of employee fatigue or of departures from the
established practices normally associated with the process. In
each case the purpose of the control chart is to detect the
change so that management may determine the cause and take
remedial action as soon as possible.

In the Figure 7.1 the process appears to be under control up to
point A, but here the persistent drift in values of sample
suggests that a change in the system has taken place.

<u>Figure 7.1 - CONTROL CHART</u>

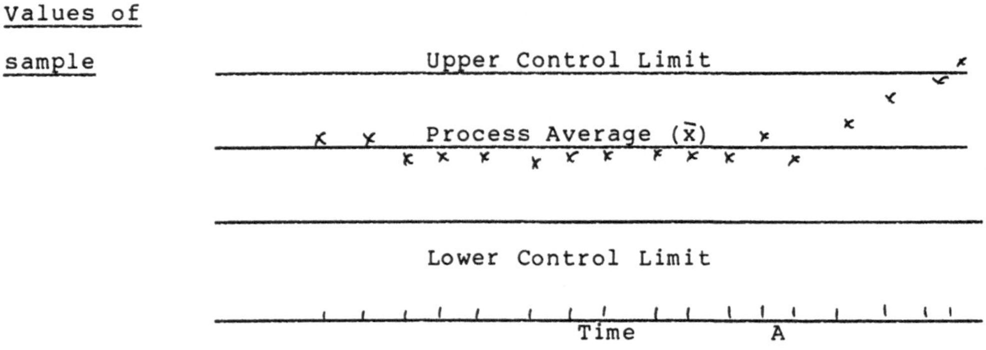

Values of

sample

It is evident that in a quality control system there is scope for
varying the control limits (by taking, for example $\mu \pm 2\sigma$, rather
than $\mu \pm 3\sigma$), and varying the frequency with which the process is
sampled. It is important that relevant control limits are set:

the control lines should separate out deviations which are usual and those which are not i.e. they should separate unassignable or chance variations and those that can be assigned to a particular cause.

(ii) $\bar{x}$ Charts

Statistical sampling theory tells us that when samples of a given (and reasonable) size are drawn from a population, the distribution of the sample means will follow the normal distribution with a mean equal to the population mean. The distribution of sample means is referred to as the sampling distribution.

Thus if one takes a number of samples from a population (and the population may or may not be normally distributed) one can expect the means of the samples to be normally distributed with a mean equal to the population mean.

We shall refer to these various parameters and statistics as follows:

μ = the population mean
x = the mean of a sample drawn from the population
σ = the population standard deviation
$S_{\bar{x}}$ = the standard deviation of a sample drawn from the population

Clearly one can now take a series of samples from the population and plot the values of the means of those samples. Because the means will be normally distributed, we can still conclude that 95% of values lie within two standard deviations of the mean. Because we are plotting values of means ($\bar{x}$), the charts are known as $\bar{x}$ charts (pronounced "x bar charts"). As the number of samples increase, the population mean, μ, mean of the sample means ($\bar{x}$) should be approximately equal. The standard deviation of the means ($s_{\bar{x}}$) will be smaller than the standard deviation of each sample because of averaging effects. It can be shown, however, that $s_{\bar{x}} = \frac{s}{\sqrt{n}}$ where n is the size of the sample.

A control chart, similar to that shown in Diagram 7.1 can be now drawn plotting the $\bar{x}$'s using $\bar{\bar{x}}$ or μ as the process average and control limits of $\pm 3s_{\bar{x}}$ or $\pm 2s_{\bar{x}}$ as appropriate.

Example 7.1

The Pathologist in charge of a large laboratory is concerned about the manual dexterity of the trainee technical officers in his laboratory. One Wednesday, he decides to ask them to pipette a twenty micro litre solution. In an attempt to obtain a fair representation of their work the task is repeated five times. The results are as follows:-

TABLE 7.1

1	2	3	4	5	6	7	8	9	10
19.8	22.4	19.5	18.3	19.6	21.2	17.9	21.6	22.1	22.6
17.5	20.9	17.2	19.1	14.2	23.8	18.6	21.2	17.2	18.4
20.1	18.4	20.4	16.8	20.8	21.9	20.6	20.1	20.1	18.7
20.9	22.5	21.3	19.6	22.6	19.8	17.0	19.6	20.5	18.2
20.6	20.9	20.8	20.2	18.8	23.0	21.2	22.4	20.6	22.9

11	12	13	14	14	16	17	18	19	20
18.1	17.6	21.7	20.3	24.3	25.5	21.0	17.8	16.3	21.8
21.0	17.9	19.9	19.2	18.4	21.7	22.6	18.8	22.3	19.2
21.9	20.6	22.5	20.3	18.7	20.0	18.7	15.7	17.1	19.8
20.6	18.2	20.5	20.7	22.0	23.1	18.9	18.4	20.8	19.9
18.4	24.4	20.8	20.8	21.4	21.4	19.0	16.2	20.2	19.9

The first step is to determine $\bar{\bar{x}}$. The sample means for the twenty samples are

    19.7 21.0 19.8 18.8 19.2 21.9 19.1 21.0 20.1 20.2
    20.0 19.7 21.1 20.2 21.0 22.4 20.0 17.4 19.3 20.1

and the mean of the mean is 20.1 i.e.

$$\bar{\bar{x}} = 20.1$$

Now $\sigma = \sqrt{\left\{ \frac{\Sigma x^2}{N} - \left(\frac{\Sigma x}{N}\right)^2 \right\}}$

$$= \sqrt{\left\{ \frac{1}{N}(19.8^2 + 17.5^2 + .. + 19.9^2) - \left(\frac{1}{N}(19.8 + 17.5 + ..19.9)\right)^2 \right\}}$$

$$= \sqrt{\frac{1}{N}(396.01 + 506.25 + ..) - \left(\frac{1}{100}(19.8 + 17.5 + ..)^2\right)}$$

$$= \sqrt{\frac{1}{100}(40793.29) - (403.969)}$$

$$= \sqrt{3.963}$$

$$= 1.99$$

Now $S_{\bar{X}} = \frac{\sigma}{\sqrt{n}}$

$$= \frac{1.99}{\sqrt{5}}$$

$$= .88$$

and hence control limits can be constructed as

$$20.1 \pm 3 \times (.88)$$

i.e. the upper control limit is 20.1 + 22.74 and the lower control limit is 20.1 - 2.64 = 17.46 and the control chart is as follows:

Figure 7.2 $\bar{x}$ CHART

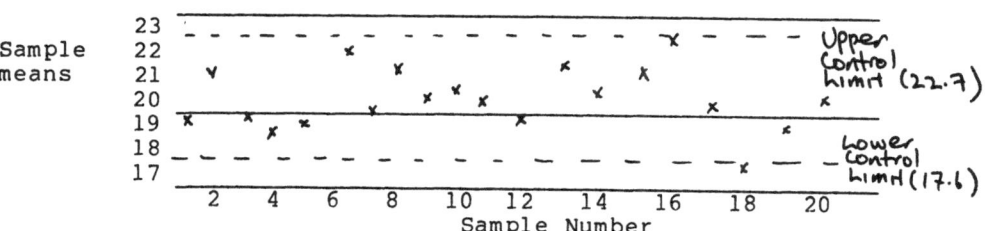

Sample means

Sample Number

As a practical matter, practitioners in the statistical control field use a short cut method for calculating control limits, using tables developed for this purpose. Such tables are provided in most operations research textbooks (see, for example, Buffa 1972). Further, as indicated above, it is quite common to calculate control charts for the <u>range</u> of each sample - these are known as R charts. The principles involved in R charts are the same as for x charts.

(iii) Control Charts for Attributes

The foregoing discussion of control charts applies in cases where a measurable variable is associated with each item of output so that $\bar{x}$ may be calculated for each sample. In many circumstances, however, only a qualitative assessment can be made, i.e. it may only be possible to characterize elements of a sample as being either acceptable or unacceptable, defective or not defective.

In each instance we can calculate that proportion or fraction of the parameter we wish to control which is unacceptable. As we are examining a dichotomy (acceptable or unacceptable) the probability distribution that is applicable in this situation is the binomial distribution. The mean p and the standard deviation S for the binomial distribution are given by:

$$\bar{p} = \frac{x}{n} = \frac{\text{number in classification}}{\text{total number observed}}$$

$$S_p = \sqrt{\frac{\bar{p}\,(1 - \bar{p})}{n}}$$

where n = the size of the subsample.

Following the general principles for control charts which we have discussed, the control limits are normally set at the process average plus and minus three standard deviations ($p \pm 3S_p$). A control chart for attributes can therefore be constructed, such a chart is commonly known as a p-chart.

Let us take as an example of the application of a p-chart the control of the number of clerical errors that occur in filing medical records. Table 7.2 shows a record of the number of errors that occurred in each of twenty samples of n = 200.

<u>TABLE 7.2</u> Record of the number of clerical errors in filing medical records (n = 200). Calculation of p and control limits shown below.

Sample Number	Number of Errors	Error Fraction	Sample Number	Number of Errors	Error Fraction
1	11	0.055	12	7	0.035
2	7	0.035	13	9	0.045
3	4	0.020	14	5	0.025
4	1	0.005	15	17	0.085
5	5	0.025	16	18	0.090
6	13	0.065	17	9	0.045
7	6	0.030	18	5	0.025
8	5	0.025	19	7	0.035
9	3	0.015	20	0	0.000
10	0	0.000	Total	131	
11	5	0.025			

For each sample the error fraction has been calculated as p = number of errors/200. The average error fraction p is calculated by summing all the errors that occurred in the combined set of 20 samples divided by the total number of observations.

Hence $\bar{p} = \dfrac{131}{20 \times 200} = 0.033$

Using the formula given above

$$S_p = \sqrt{\frac{\bar{p}(1-\bar{p})}{n}}$$

$$= \sqrt{\frac{.033(1-0.033)}{200}}$$

$$= \sqrt{\frac{.033 \times .967}{200}}$$

$$= .0126$$

$$\therefore 3S_p = .038$$

Thus Upper Control Limit = $\bar{p} + 3S_p$ = .033 + .038 = .071
and Lower Control Limit = $\bar{p} - 3S_p$ = .033 - .038 = 0

The resultant control chart is shown in Figure 7.3.

Figure 7.3 p-Chart for clerical errors in medical record filing

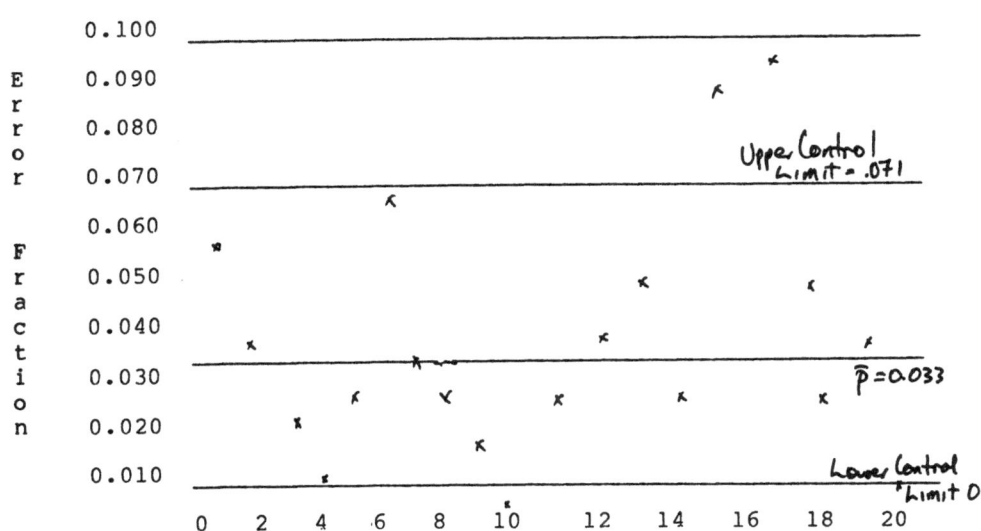

Note that samples 15 and 16 fall above the upper control limit. In this instance, investigation showed that at the time of those two samples construction work in the office was going on to remodel part of the area. Apparently the confusion and noise had affected the accuracy of the employee doing the filing, and this was regarded as an assignable cause of variation. In establishing the process average and the control limits for further observations, we would eliminate these 2 samples from our data to calculate a revised process average and control limits.

(iv) Control Charts for Defects

Sometimes the parameter to be controlled cannot be expressed as a simple proportion such as was true with p charts. In weaving, for example, the number of defects per 10 square yards of material might be the parameter to be controlled. In such instances, each defect is in itself minor, but a large number of defects per unit might be objectionable. The probability distribution commonly applicable in this situation is the Poisson distribution. In the Poisson distribution the standard deviation s is equal to the square root of the mean value, $\bar{c}$. The result is that the calculation of control limits is extremely simple:

Upper Control Limit = $\bar{c} + 3\sqrt{\bar{c}}$
Lower Control Limit = $\bar{c} - 3\sqrt{\bar{c}}$

Alternatively, control limits can be calculated by direct calculation of poisson probabilities and examination of the cumulative likelihood of an event. There are many parameters within hospitals, particularly those which relate to unexpected results of the medical care process, which conform to the criteria of the Poisson process. Briefly stated, these criteria are for independence of each occurrence from all other occurrences, a low probability of occurrence and an equal probability of an occurrence in any given small time period. Many kinds of accidental occurrences, such as accidents occurring to staff members, accidents occurring to guests and visitors to the hospital, patient falls, and medication errors may be expected to follow a Poisson process. In addition, it is possible that certain employee turnover statistics follow a Poisson process, and that at least certain forms of patient death statistics, particularly those where the risk of death is usually small, are Poisson. (A given statistic can be tested for the closeness of a Poisson approximation using the chi-square goodness of fit test.)

The following record of receipt of unusual incidents reports occurring to patients will illustrate. Each day r reports are received. The values are listed in chronological order in columns.

TABLE 7.3 NUMBER OF INCIDENT REPORTS EACH DAY

Month 1			Month 2		
2	2	3	5	3	7
3	6	0	4	2	5
1	6	3	4	1	5
2	2	2	2	7	3
3	3	5	3	1	5
4	1	6	5	3	2
4	4	8	4	0	4
1	4	4	6	5	1
2	2	9	4	3	2
3	4	1	2	5	3
		3			

The control limits can be calculated by use of the mean and standard deviation method or directly from the Poisson distribution.

1) Over the 61 day period, a total of 209 reports were received.

$$\bar{c} = \frac{209}{61}$$

$$= 3.42$$

$$\sqrt{\bar{c}} = 1.845$$

and hence 99% Upper Control Limit $= \bar{c} + 3\sqrt{\bar{c}}$

$$= 3.42 + 3 \times 1.845$$

$$= 8.95$$

99% Lower Control Limit $= \bar{c} - 3\sqrt{\bar{c}}$

$$= 3.42 - 3 \times 1.845$$

$$= 0$$

2) Alternatively we could consider the occurrence of the incident report as a Poisson process. Table 7.3 shows the actual distribution of incident reports, the relative probabilities and the probabilities associated with a Poisson process with mean of 3.4

TABLE 7.4 FREQUENCY OF REPORTS

r	Frequency	Relative Frequency	Poisson Probability = 3.4
0	2	.0328	.0334
1	7	.1148	.1135
2	12	.1968	.1929
3	13	.2132	.2186
4	11	.1804	.1858
5	8	.1312	.1264
6	4	.0656	.0716
7	2	.0328	.0348
8	1	.0164	.0148
9	1	.0164	.0056
10	0	0	.0019
11	0	0	.0006
12	0	0	.0002
	$\overline{16}$		

$$\text{Mean} = \left\{ (2 \times 0) + (7 \times 1) + (2 \times 12) + (3 \times 13) + (4 \times 11) + (5 \times 8) + (6 \times 4) + (7 \times 2) + (8 \times 1) + (9 \times 1) + (10 \times 0) + (11 \times 0) + (12 \times 0) \right\} / 61$$

$$= \frac{0 + 7 + 24 + 39 + 44 + 40 + 24 + 14 + 8 + 9 + 0 + 0 + 0}{61}$$

$$= 3.42$$

The appropriateness of the use of the Poisson distribution can be checked by using the chi-square goodness of fit test, which shows the difference is not significant at the 5% level. Table 7.5 shows the cumulative probabilities for the Poisson distribution.

TABLE 7.5 CUMULATIVE PROBABILITIES OF POISSON DISTRIBUTION, $\lambda = 3.4$

r	Cumulative Probability
0	.0334
1	.1469
2	.3398
3	.5584
4	.7442
5	.8706
6	.9422
7	.9770
8	.9918
9	.9974
10	.9993
11	.9999
12	1.0000

Hence at r = 8 the cumulative probability is .99 and thus r = 8 should be used as the 99% Upper Control Limit (with 0 as the Lower Control Limit).

As the population at risk under a Poisson process become larger, the mean or expected value increases. Values of the Poisson formula are not tabulated for larger means, but the distribution approximates the normal distribution. Use of the normal distribution to set control limits is usual for expected values greater than 25 and introduces no significant error in the control system.

APPLICATIONS TO HEALTH ADMINISTRATION

Statistical quality control techniques can be used by management in a number of areas to draw attention to situations where there is a significant deviation from the normal. A manager, for example, cannot be concerned with the waiting time of every single patient in the emergency room. If, however, that waiting time stretches so that it is, on average, 5 hours per patient, management should be involved. Similarly, the Chief Laboratory Technician does not check every test performed in a laboratory but rather concentrates on unusual tests etc.

These are examples of management by exception whereby only exceptions from the norm are reported and acted upon. This "filtering" of reporting highlights for management attention areas which are malfunctioning or where specific action is required.

Statistical quality control is one technique management can use to highly exceptional occurrences. Management can have their attention drawn to circumstances or events which are 'out of control'. The $\bar{x}$ chart, for example has specified 'control limits' and when these are exceeded action by management is usually warranted.

Examples of applications of quality control abound in hospitals but three will suffice.

(1) **Service Departments: Laboratories and Food Preparation**

Quality control in laboratories has been part of routine operations for many years. Most hospital laboratories regularly sample the output of automated analyses to ensure that readings and results provided to clinicians are accurate. There is an extensive literature on these uses of quality control techniques (e.g. see Whitehead 1977).

Management will obviously be interested in fluctuations in the standard of food prepared for patients. Thus measures of temperature, number of calories, time of arrival in the wards, bacterial count etc. could be made. These results could be plotted on a control chart and when values are greater or less than previously determined control limits, investigations and reports would be required.

How often does a manager hear, for example, that the food is always cold yet the catering officer will answer that on that day a machine broke down or a member of staff was away etc. etc. If the process is out of control every day there must be something wrong with the whole system!

(2) Volume of Services

Several different types of services within a hospital or ambulatory clinic can have quite substantial fluctuations in their availability or utilisation. Thus the number of patients attending a clinic may fluctuate around 30 except when the medical practitioner is on holiday. Similarly, the number of cleaners on duty in a particular area may fluctuate around 20. Management will want to know when the number of cleaners on duty is critically short or the number of patients attending the clinics are at a point which overtaxes the system. Again control charts can be used.

Historical data will exist from which to calculate the mean and standard deviation and having calculated these, daily variations can be recorded. Again management will quickly see occasions when there is a shortage of cleaners or an excess of patients attending clinics.

(3) Quality of Care

The evaluation of patient care provides an opportunity for some of the most interesting and important applications of statistical quality control techniques. In an area fraught with vague definitions and hazy objectives it is not to be expected that the introduction of quantitative techniques will be simple and universally acceptable. Nevertheless a number of systems have been developed which attracted considerable supported and were implemented in a number of hospitals.

(i) Quality of nursing care

The Commission for Administrative Services in Hospitals (CASH) has developed a system for nursing care appraisal (see Commission for Administrative Services in Hospitals, 1965. The system has also be described in Griffith, 1972).

The primary objectives of the system are as follows:

1. To provide a measure which will indicate the level of the quality of care and services; the degree of nursing proficiency.

2. To provide such measures on a continuing basis as a vital on going management control.

3. To provide feedback in order to allow the necessary corrective action.

4. To provide a means of establishing staffing patterns based on optimum personnel utilisation and assured quality of care and service.

The Commission points out that three rules must be used to ensure a valid use of statistical quality control techniques:

1. Samples (in this case patients, rooms and charts) must be selected at random.

2. A sufficient number of samples (observations) must be taken.

3. An affirmative or negative decision regarding the attribute being observed must truly represent the immediate condition.

The system is based on checking three major areas:-

1. The patient and his or her immediate environs. (The patient environment includes patient welfare and safety, patient comfort and the patient's room.)

2. The patient chart.

3. The nursing unit.

A system of additional checks has been developed to increase the statistical validity of the system and to ensure that an appropriate number of observations are made.

An index, based on the weighted sum of the three major areas, is calculated and plotted on a control chart. The Commission has recommended that the quality index be charted on the same chart as utilisation figures.

The questionnaires used in the CASH system have been evaluated by a number of authors (see, for example, Smith, 1972) and although the sections of the questionnaire on housekeeping and nursing unit related activities were found to yield sensitive and reliable indicators, the more clinically related sections were found to be poor discriminators. Levine and Kahn (1975) point out:-

"Several conceptual approaches to the assessment of quality of (nursing) care have been suggested and some have been tried; to date, very little progress has been made in the development of a useful tool for quality measurement."

However, that conclusion is overly pessimistic. More and more hospitals (and other health facilities) are recognsing the value of standardised quality measurement techniques both because of the direct benefit and use that nursing managers (and staff) can make of the results but also because of the requirements of accrediting agencies. Statistical quality control techniques will play an increasing role in these efforts.

(ii) Quality of Medical Care

Increasing attention is also being paid to methods of clinical review or medical audit: most involve some form of identification of abnormal occurrences and many involve statistical quality control techniques. Many systems, for example, highlight results which are statistically significantly different from a mean or standard value.

Although recent developments in quality assurance have tended to deemphasise routine on-going monitoring (e.g. see Skillicorn, 1980), statistical quality control techniques still play a major role in monitoring medical care. Barnett and others (1978), for example, developed a computer based quality assurance program relying on information collected as part of the routine patient care recording process. As the system was a supplement to an onging data collection, the additional expense involved in developing the computer based quality assurance component was minimised.

Organisations involved in monitoring health insurance claims (including PSROs), make extensive use of statistical quality control techniques. Rosenberg et al (1976) have described a system used as part of the New York City Medicare Program. Under that system control limits are set to identify statistically deviant or undesirable practices who are then subjected to further detailed examination.

Many other systems, such as the PAS/QAM system developed by the Commission on Professional and Hospital Activities use similar methods.

CONCLUSION

The concept of statistical quality control represents the epitome of management by exception. Limits based on probabilities are set so that random variations, due to uncontrollable chance causes, are ignored. When a deviation that is larger than expected occurs, however, control limits signal this fact immediately and call into play a corrective procedure. The result is that managerial personnel do not waste their time on the random variations, but their attention is called immediately to those situations where the probability is high that a real change in the process being controlled has occurred.

As has been pointed out, the selection of a control plan involves a balance between the cost of investigation and the cost of letting a process continue that is out of control. The three factors which influence these costs and which may be set by the designer of the control system are the control limits, the sample size, and the interval between samples. Although it is not common to set the levels of these three factors by a careful investigation, models have been developed which have this objective.

Finally, although the basic ideas and procedures for statistical control have been developed in a framework for industrial quality control, we should recognize that the principles are broadly applicable to the control of any parameter which can be measured and sample. Thus, whereas initial applications were in the field of statistical quality control, it is becoming much more common to find the use of these methods in work measurement, cost control, control of labor turnover, absenteeism, and so on.

REFERENCES

Ackoff, R.L. & Sasieni, M.W. (1968) Fundamentals of Operations Research Wiley.

Barnett, C.O., Winicoff, R., Dorsey, J.L., Morgan, M.M. & Lurie, R.S. (1978) Quality Assurance Through Automated Monitoring & Concurrent Feedback using a Computer-based Medical Information System Medical Care Vol XVI No 1, November, pp.962-971.

Commission for Administrative Services in Hospitals (1965) A Quality Control Plan for Nursing Service, The Commission. (Available in Abstracts of Hospital Management Studies, Microfilm reel 160, NU1054.)

Griffith, J.R. (1972) Quantitative Techniques for Hospital Planning & Control, Lexington.

Huitson, A. & Keen, J. (1965) Essentials of Quality Control, Heinemann.

Levine, E. & Kahn, H.D. Health Manpower Models in Shuman, L.J., Speas, R.D. & Young, J.P. (eds) (1975) Operations Research in Health Care, John Hopkins University Press.

Rosenberg, S.N., Gunston, C., Beneson, L. & Klein, A. (1976) An Eclectic Approach to Quality Control in Fee for Service Health Care: The New York City Medicaid Experience American Journal of Public Health, 66:21-30 January.

Simmons, D.A. Patient Care & Support in Simmons, D.A. (ed) (1972) Medical & Hospital Control Systems, Little Brown.

Skillicorn, S.A. (1980) Quality & Accountability: A New Era in American Hospitals, Edit Consulting Inc.

Smith, R.L. (1972) Analysis of the CASH-type Nursing Quality Instrument, unpublished paper, Bureau of Hospital Administration, University of Michigan.

Whitehead, T.P. (1977) Advances in Quality Control Advances in Clinical Chemistry, vol 19, pp.175-205.

Wild, R. (1972) Management & Production, Penguin.

SEARCH - SUMMARY

Search problems use properties of statistical distributions to implement management by exception.

The basic principles are implemented by control charts. We plot the values of various elements on the chart to discover whether the values fall into an acceptable range. The "elements" plotted may vary, most commonly they could be:

(i)   single values of an element sampled
(ii)   values of the mean of a small sample
(iii) values of certain attribute (e.g. percentage defective)
(iv)   numbe of defects found.

In addition we might plot the range of a sample.

(i) Single values

Here we assume that the population we are sampling from is normally distributed. The process average is the population mean, the control limits are based on the population standard deviation. We plot the actual values on the chart.

(ii) Means

We use the property that the means of samples follow a normal distribution and plot those means on a control chart. The standard deviation of the samples is used to calculate the control limits.

(iii) Attributes

Where only qualitative assessments can be made, a mean is inappropriate. We thus use the binomial theorem to derive the process average and the standard deviation.

(iv) Defects

We use the poisson distribution in those cases where we can calculate the number of defects but cannot express it as a proportion. The standard deviation of a Poisson distribution is equal to the square root of the mean and we either use this fact, or poisson tables, to derive our control chart.

8   CONCLUSION

A central theme so far has been stress on the need to evaluate the assumptions underlying applications of operations research for all such studies make assumptions and some are more realistic than others.

It is up to you, as a current or prospective health service manager to evaluate these applications. The questions involved will occur time and time again:

> What is the problem being solved?
> How have the authors (or consultants) modelled or simplified it?
> What assumptions have they made?
> How realistic are those assumptions?
> What other models could have been developed?
> What other assumptions could have been made?

The application of operations research will always involve judgements: which model will be used in this situation? do we assume the trend in the last 2 years will continue? what difference is made if we assume the trend in the last 5 years?

Operations researchers have a number of techniques for resolving dilemmas such as these. Good operations research studies will be written in clear english, highlighting the implications of the decisions that are to be made, with some sensitivity testing of the outcomes. Further, good studies will reveal the assumptions that are involved in the model; in the data used etc. Obviously, not all studies can be as thorough as we would like. There may well be a place for the "quick and dirty" study to provide the administrator with some quick pseudo-answers, but the analyst involved should highlight the shortcuts that have been made and the possibilities of error.

Beware the Snake Oil Salesmen

Operations research and mathematical models are not magic tools, which will provide the health administrator and planner with a panacea, despite the claims that are sometimes made by the more naive promoters. More insidiously, operations research can be a tool in the fights for power within and between organisations. Planning agencies, government bureaucracies and other hospitals may employ "consultants" to devise reports favourable to their position. The techniques are legion but some of the more common are:

(a) Mathematicisation

A common way to force the determined administrator off the
scent is to mathematicise i.e. lapse into complex
mathematical formulae that are either completely
unintelligible or sufficiently forebidding to daunt all but
the hardiest. This approach can be used to obscure
assumptions or important (and weak) leaps in the argument.

(b) Obfuscation

A second technique, often used in association with
mathematicisation is obfuscation (according to the
dictionary: darken, obscure, confuse, bewilder). Although
this is probably most easily done by use of technical
jargon, tortuous reasoning and "methodological appendixes"
can assist.

(c) Oraculation

Most health workers who will come in contact with operations
research studies are employed in bureaucracies, hospitals,
planning agencies etc.   "Authorities" and oracles
(dictionary definition: Person or thing serving as
infallible, though mysterious, guide, test or indicator;
authoritative, profoundly wise) may be relied upon to give
weight to the opinion expressed in the document. Only
occasionally is there a "slip up" when, for instance, two
conflicting oracular pronouncements are quoted.

(d) Statisculation

The experienced consultant is able to use the full range of
statistical techniques designed to ensure acceptance of
their report. Huff (1973) provides a good overview of
these. Techniques such as the Gee-Whiz Graph, the carefully
chosen definition may be used.

(e) Ceteris paribus

One favourite technique is to mention a long list of
assumptions or conditions (thus exhausting the readers) and
then assert the conclusions, ceretis paribus. (Dictionary
definition: other things being equal).   Hopefully the
reader will not be able to recall what has been left out nor
will be able to comprehend the horrendous occurrences or
conditions which are being assumed away.

(f) Spurious Sensitivities

The truly accomplished writer will undertake a spurious
sensitivity test. Sensitivity testing normally involves
assessing how 'sensitive' the solution is to changes in the
values of relevant variables. An experienced "operations
researcher" can include sensitivity tests on variables which
indeed cause relatively little change, thus drawing
attention away from variables which include just as many
assumptions but are critical.

(g) Elimination

At the bottom of the barrel of tricks is elimination.
Simply ignore, not mention or eliminate doubtful areas or
shaky premises. Taken in conjunction with a bulky (and well
presented) document and a majestic (or magical) sweep of the
hand, even the most crucial assumptions can remain
unmentioned and hence unnoticed.

These "dirty tricks" are just that and should not be used to
condemn good, well designed operations research studies.

However, many experienced health administrators and operations
researchers are now increasingly sceptical of the use of
operations research in health services, despite the fact that
mathematical modelling and operations research has a lot to
offer. The hunches and traditions upon which many decisions are
being made are normally inadequate. With the rapid escalation in
health expenditure, government and other third party payers will
increasingly seek justification of new services, buildings and
equipment and, hopefully, decision makers will look askance at
woolly generalisations. Similarly one hopes that hospital boards
and funding agencies will be critical of baldly stated requests
with no attached justification.

In an area such as health administration, administrators and
decision makers are susceptible to emotional pleas and moral
blackmail and requests for statistically valid justifications are
shrugged off. But the efficacy of modern medical techniques are
increasingly questioned and administrators have an obligation to
ensure that investments in new equipment will return dividends in
terms of improved patient care, shorter length of stay, improved
accuracy of diagnosis (provided it is associated with an improved
prognosis) etc.

As Parker (1978) argues:

"Policy problems in the health and public sectors are
quickly assuming a new level of complexity. Thus, the
health/public sector analyst is being confronted with
the task of identifying, formulating, evaluating, and
making choices among larger and more complicated sets
of decision alternatives. Given the context of such
decisions, less-than-effective choices could adversely
affect the health and social well-being of whole
sections of a population. What seems to be needed,
therefore, is an approach that would provide system and
objectivity to the policy-making process. The use of
quantitative techniques, so long applied to problems in
the private and industrial sectors, would be the
mainstay of such an approach."

Operations Research can be used

It is not inevitable that health applications of operations
research will follow "the basic pattern of grand pretensions,
faulty execution, and puny results" (Elmore, 1978). The recent
literature has included reports of a number of "successful"
studies (see, for example, the collection in Boldy (1981) or the
reports carried regularly in the journal, Interfaces). In
addition as Morris (1982) points out:

"What goes unrecognized is that the health services can
and do implement the findings of appreciable numbers of
crude studies of the 'bucket arithmetic' type. While
usually quite unsuitable for presentation to learned
societies or publication in learned journals, such
quantitative analyses are nowadays an integral part of
routine health service management and development.
Introspective concern with the disappointments of
complex OR does little justice to a large volume of
useful, if simple, studies. There is an undoubted need
for 'pure' OR, in the same way as there is a need for
'pure' epidemiology or 'pure' management theory.
However, like epidemiology and management theory, OR
will not realize its optimum impact if it is perceived
as the exclusive and arcane preserve of a sophisticated
elite, its boundaries delineated from within."

Interestingly, Haro (1977) has suggested that there is a
decreasing importance of formal publication in most areas of
health statistics. Further, increasing attention is being
devoted to implementation of operations research both generally
(Huysmans, 1970; Schultz & Slevin, 1975; Doktor et al, 1979) and
in the health system (Lagergren, 1981).

The tools in the operations researcher's kit bag (some of which
have been outlined in the preceding pages) can assist health
system managers and planners.

As Helmer et al (1982) note:

"It is not essential for a hospital administrator to
possess the mathematical knowledge to transfer a
management problem into computer language or
mathematical programs in order to obtain a solution.

Operations researchers and medical system engineers
have been trained for this task. However, to assure
the successful application of management science
techniques, the administrator must have the ability to
recognize a problem which can be solved by management
science techniques and to help formulate a model to
resolve it. Formulation of such a model, as we have
stated, is an important aspect of applying management
science techniques. It is here that the expertise,
judgment, and creativity of the administrator are
critical."

They go on to argue that the administrator must therefore have
the following skills:

"1. The ability to recognize hospital or health care
management situations in which management science
might be used effectively.

2. The ability to communicate effectively with a
technical specialist to explain the nature of the
problem and the results desired.

   3. The ability to understand the results of management
      science studies so that the full value of the
      information and alternatives are fully
      appreciated."

To this we might add the ability to understand the assumptions
that are likely to have been made and thus, to be prepared to
question the report as presented.

The overall objective of these notes has been to enhance your
abilities in those areas.   Good luck in using them!

REFERENCES

Boldy, D. (ed) (1981) Operational Research Applied to Health Services, Croom Helm.

Doktor, R., Schultz, R.L. & Slevin, D.P. (eds) (1979) The Implementation of Management Science, (TIMS Studies in the Management Sciences Vol. 13) North Holland.

Elmore, R.F. (1978) "Organisational Models of Social Program Implementation", Public Policy, Vol. 26, No. 2, pp.185-228.

Haro, A.S. (1977) "Health Information Systems", Proceedings of the Royal Society of Medicine, Vol. 70, October, pp.701-708.

Helmer, F.T., Kuchemar, W.H., Oppermann, E.B. & Suver, J.D. (1982) "Basic Management Science Techniques for Decision Analysis", Hospital & Health Service Administration, Vol. 27, No.2, March-April, pp.58-71.

Huff, D. (1973) How to Lie with Statistics, Penguin.

Huysmans, J. (1970) The Implementation of Operations Research, Wiley.

Parker, B.R. (1978) "Quantitative Decision Techniques for the Health/Public Sector Decision Maker: An Analysis and Classification of Resources", Journal of Health Politics, Policy and Law, Vol. 3, No. 3, pp.388-417.

Lagergren, M. (1981) Implementation of O.R. Projects in Health Care in Boldy, D. (ed) (1981) Operational Research Applied to Health Services, Croom Helm.

Morris, D. (1982) Book Review in Community Medicine, Vol. 4, No. 2, pp.147-148.

Schultz, R.L. & Slevin, D.P. (eds) (1975) Implementing Operations Research/Management Science, American Elsevier.

Lecture Notes in Medical Informatics